Introduction

Physical or Hatha Yoga is the most complete exercise system in the world. It mobilises joints, keeps the back amazingly flexible and tones every muscle, helping you to find the best body shape for your individual height and build and keeping that *Fabulous Shape Forever!* As the exercises are combined with slow, deep breathing it also helps you relax at will, conquer stress and sleep well. It is a complete system of positive health that you can do in your own time at your own pace and with no financial investment whatsoever.

Yoga works on the entire body releasing tensions and toning every single part of the body but it does much more than that as you practice. You start to feel better, to trust your own judgement, to cope with life's troubles much more easily and, gradually, you develop your own unique potential and achieve self realisation.

HOW I CAME TO YOGA

After leaving school I trained as a State Registered Nurse at St Mary's Hospital, Paddington. In my first year I earned £2 per week, admittedly our full board, lodging and laundry was paid for by the hospital, but it was 1960. I was eighteen, London was swinging and you can't swing much on £2 per week. So to supplement my meagre earnings I joined a modelling agency and a baby-sitting agency and managed to work in my off-duty hours. This meant my hours were long and I was frequently exhausted with no time or energy to enjoy myself.

As my training progressed I moved to a hospital department called 'the Metabolic Unit', where I found myself helping the doctors discover and treat problems and diseases caused by nutritional deficiencies and diet problems in general. I adored this work and bought every book I could find on diet and nutrition.

One particularly late evening I handed some test results to a doctor and we discussed more dietary changes for the patient as our current treatment was not working. As we talked, the doctor looked at me and said that if only we all ate just *natural foods* in their *natural state* a lot of dietary problems could be eliminated. The words hit home. I began to think about my own eating pattern of rushed snacks between increasingly exhausting schedules and realised that I had been studying nutrition, thinking about the patients' problems and had never even considered myself. I had a problem remaining slim enough for my modelling jobs and had felt the answer to my tired skin was in creams that I was not able to afford. But the doctor's words made me think, so I eliminated all biscuits, cakes, sweets and packaged goods and concentrated on water, fresh fruits, juices, salads, fresh vegetables, a little chicken, fish, cheese and meat. I was lucky at St Mary's as the food for the staff was very good, with a wide selection of lovely salads and fruits available around the clock. In one month the change was amazing. My tiredness went and I lost weight, even though I was eating much more. I started to feel really well, in fact so well I never wanted to go back to my old eating habits. My skin improved, my nails became strong and altogether I looked and felt at my best.

After finishing my nursing training, I learned three languages and then joined British Airways (then BOAC) as an air stewardess. I still kept to my natural food plan and found that no matter where I was in the world it was really easy to stick to and my sense of well being just got better and better.

After leaving my flying job I got married and moved to Scotland and had two children in two and a half years.

The contrast of being a free spirit and flying around the world to being home in Scotland with two small children was quite considerable, to say the least, and I began to feel restless. My body was in need of toning after the birth of my second child, so I searched for an exercise class to firm it up a bit. It was solely with this in mind that I found a Yoga class, and one damp and dreary Monday morning walked into the class for my first lesson. I could not believe my eyes. The teacher was in her late fifties but was as agile as a child and had the body of an eighteen year old. She radiated energy and a genuine *joie de vivre*. I also couldn't believe how appallingly stiff I was. Since giving up flying, where I was used to swimming in the Caribbean, water skiing and the like, I had done practically no exercise – and my body really showed it.

I remember thinking that Frankie Lindsay, the teacher, must have been born flexible and was obviously double-jointed and that I had been born with different joints and was naturally stiff. Frankie was quick to explain that this was not so. My body had stiffened because I had not used it properly and it would be just as flexible as hers if I came to one class a week. I did just that – and did two classes a week when possible.

Frankie had arrived in Scotland from America, where she had been taught by Richard Hittleman whose books and television programmes were huge successes, both here and in the USA.

Word spread fast about Frankie's classes and it soon became obvious that she needed help to cope with the huge demand. So she started a three-year teacher training scheme and that was the start of the West of Scotland Yoga Teachers' Association. I was lucky to be able to take this course and thoroughly enjoyed it. The benefits were amazing. My body became better toned and

barbara currie's
YOGA
workout

having a fabulous shape forever

INDEX

I would especially like to thank Louise Dixon at André Deutsch for her tremendous hard work, amazing stamina and delightful sense of humour during the editing and re-editing of this book. It has been a joy to work with her. My thanks also to Claire Proctor for typing the manuscript and meeting all the deadlines with a smile on her face; to the book's designer, Linda Wade, for her wonderful work; to Roger Dixon for his beautiful photographs (and the kindness and patience he showed while I assumed positions he had never seen before!); to Panilla Marott for lovely make-up in impossible positions; and to Maureen Corgiolu for making my beautiful leotards.

Many thanks also to my husband Gordon, my children Lysanne and Mark, my mother Babs and my brother Richard, for the love, support and encouragement they always give me.

Please note: not all exercises are suitable for everyone and this or any other programme may result in injury or illness. To reduce the risk to you, please consult your doctor before the beginning of this exercise programme. The instructions and advice presented are in no way intended as a substitute for medical guidance.

The writer and publishers of this book do not accept any responsibility for any injury or accident incurred as a result of following this exercise programme.

First published in Great Britain in 1997 by Chameleon Books, an imprint of André Deutsch Limited
Paperback edition published in 2002 by André Deutsch Limited,
an imprint of the Carlton Publishing Group
20 Mortimer Street, London W1T 3JW
This edition published in 2002 for Index Books Ltd

A catalogue record for this book is available from the British Library

ISBN 0 233 05031 0

Printed in Italy

more flexible than it had ever been, my energy levels increased tremendously and I felt really great.

On completion of my training, my husband's business interests meant that we had to move back to the London area, where I searched in vain for a Yoga class. I took it for granted that Frankie Lindsay's was typical of all Yoga classes, but nothing was further from the truth. I missed Frankie's warm smile, her energy and her genuine desire to help. In her classes there was always a wonderful atmosphere, lots of laughter and delight when a student managed to do a previously unobtainable position. I could not find this anywhere.

Then one day in the hall next to my daughter's school, I saw a Yoga class advertised. Ideal! – I could drop the children off, do the class, shop and then collect the children again. I joined the class and at the end of the first lesson the teacher pointed a finger at me and said 'You are a trained Yoga teacher, aren't you? Will you take over the class as of next week? I am leaving for Sweden!'

I was really taken aback, no way did I want to start my own class, as my house and children were not yet organised and I had a lot to do. But the other class members insisted and so my classes started.

That was twenty-five years ago and over the years I have learned an amazing amount from my pupils. I have witnessed many people becoming totally rejuvenated by Yoga. All my pupils love the energy and feeling of well being it gives them and the beautiful lean body shape and excellent posture. I have taught many thousands of people in my time and am now delighted to have the opportunity of teaching you.

WHAT IS YOGA?

The word Yoga means the union of the body, mind and spirit.

The Yogis of ancient India had a tremendous understanding of how the body, mind and spirit were interconnected and for total health must work together harmoniously, a feeling that we find very difficult to understand in the West.

The origins of Yoga date back well before the birth of Christ. In fact, traces of Yoga postures have been found in ruins dating back to 5000 BC. We first find Yoga mentioned in the *Vedas* (3000-1200 BC). The *Upanishads* were later, about 800 BC and the *Bhagavad Gita* was written about 500 BC. The Classical Yoga system, the *Yoga Sutras*, were written by Patanjali in about 200 BC. We are then told that the Goddess Parvati prayed for the solution to all human suffering. In a dream, Lord Siva revealed to her the greatest of all sciences for the perfect physical and mental development of mankind, the science of Hatha Yoga! This was then handed down from guru (teacher) to pupil. Then, in the sixteenth century, the *Hatha Yoga Pradipika* was written down by Swami Svatmarama and is the classic work on Hatha, or Physical Yoga. Since then, Yoga has been traditionally handed from teacher to pupil and now Hatha Yoga is the most practiced form of Yoga in the West.

Other forms of Yoga are:
- Raja Yoga, the Yoga of the mind
- Karma Yoga, the Yoga of Action
- Bhakti Yoga, the Yoga of Devotion
- Jnana Yoga, the Yoga of the Intellect

HATHA YOGA

Hatha Yoga comprises amazing physical exercises that work every single area in the body. This is combined with balancing postures, brilliant breathing techniques and relaxation. All these work together to get the body into the best physical state possible, leaving the mind calm, clear and relaxed, to help the student achieve his or her own unique potential.

Who Can Do Yoga?

Anyone. My pupils range between age five and 85, and as long as you go gently without strain, Yoga is for you. *Do remember*, however, that Yoga is for healthy people. If you have had an accident or injury or are pregnant, have just had a baby or any illness or have any concerns about your health whatsoever, you must obtain your doctor's consent before you begin.

How Do I Start?

I have divided this book into ten Lessons. Simply start with Lesson One and do it to your own ability, without strain. Stay with this Lesson for as long as it takes to feel comfortable with it, then do Lesson Two. Again, stay with Lesson Two for as long as it takes to feel comfortable in the movements and then alternate Lessons One and Two and, when you are comfortable with both, move on at your own pace to Lesson Three, and so on.

Keep going in this way so that eventually you are alternating all ten Lessons. You will then possess an exercise system that will help you to radiate health and have a *Fabulous Shape Forever.*

When is the Best Time To Practice?

This depends on you. All our lives are different. I personally find it easier to exercise first thing in the morning. I love early mornings and it is supposed to be the best time for exercise. However, I have friends who would hate this idea. These people come to life in the evening and prefer to exercise then.

If you like to vary your time of day that's OK, but your body does like to get used to a regular time of day if possible.

If you are really pushed for time, try to do Lesson One's Ten-Minute Miracle (see pp12-20) every morning of the working week and maybe at the weekend try another Lesson. All the other Lessons will take about 20-30 minutes, but the six postures in Lesson One are a fabulous exercise routine on their own. As you learn Yoga, it will become automatic to stretch on waking, to breath slowly and deeply if you start to feel stressed, to give yourself time to just BE, to do the chest expansion when your neck starts to tighten, and so on. Gradually it will become a way of life.

How Often Should I Practice?

Again this is up to you. Ideally it would be wonderful if you could do a whole lesson per day. Little and often is much more beneficial to your body than a lot once a week but I know this can be difficult and that is why I have made Lesson One much shorter. Try to do Lesson One, or the Salute to the Sun from Lesson Five (see pp68-72) when you are comfortable with, it every day and then spend your time on the other Lessons as your schedule permits – at least three times a week, if possible. Don't feel guilty if you miss for a few days, but do start again quickly.

YOGA FOR YOUR HEALTH

As Yoga improves general health, students frequently tell me that certain conditions which were once a real worry to them gradually disappear.

Yoga works because it is releasing tension from every part of the body. The sense of relaxation felt after a class is caused because the entire body has been carefully worked – inhaling deeply, exhaling slowly, stretching every muscle to eliminate tension and stimulating blood flow with the final relaxation ensuring that your entire body is comfortable.

The specific movements for particular parts of the body help, of course, but it is your half hour or ten minutes a day that are really doing the work. That's why, even on your hectic days, you should try to do Lesson One or Salute to the Sun when you can manage it.

Although Yoga is extremely beneficial for your health, it must never be used as a substitute for your doctor's treatment. You are your doctor's patient, he or she is advising you and aiding your recovery and sometimes their treatment might conflict with your Yoga exercises. Ask your doctor's advice and, if necessary, show him this book and the movements you are proposing to do and obtain his permission before embarking on certain movements. (Please note: your doctor's permission and advice must be obtained if you have had an accident or injury, if you have recently had surgery, if you are pregnant or have just had a baby, if you are overweight, have very high blood pressure or heart disease, or if you have any concerns about your health and your suitability to exercise whatsoever.)

There are various health problems that Yoga can help with. Here is a list of some of them and the movements that can be most beneficial.

Arthritis and Rheumatism

I have found that Yoga exercises can help these conditions tremendously. However, please go carefully and never strain.

Lesson One, practiced every morning, helps the spine and Yoga's gentle movements can help to mobilise the joints. Remember never to strain any joint and make sure that you relax for at least ten minutes every day.

Back Problems

The Yoga belief is that the spine must be moved carefully in all directions – forwards, backwards, up, side to side and twisted in both directions to create a healthy spine and thus a healthy nervous system. That is why Lesson One's stretches are so good. Go at your own pace, without strain, and simply persevere – gradually you will become more mobile. If you can, find a qualified Yoga teacher to guide and help you. All backs are different and you will need constant encouragement to help you through your difficult days.

Asthma and Breathing Difficulties

Yoga can be very helpful for asthmatics. Try to do Lesson One every morning. Learn the Complete Breath from Lesson Two (see p22) and the Alternate Nostril Breathing Exercise from Lesson Six (see p87). Learn to relax. Every night before bed do the Pose of a Fish from Lesson Six (see p94), this helps to relieve tension from the chest. Concentrate on the Backwards Bends – the Cobra, the Bow, the Camel and the Wheel – as these are very good for relieving tightness and expanding the chest.

Again, do obtain your doctor's permission and try to find a qualified teacher to help you.

Tension, Stress and Headaches

Learning to combat tension with the Complete Breath (see p22) and the Alternate Nostril Breathing Exercise (see p87) will help you tremendously. During your day, try to stop at intervals and consciously check your body over to see if you are doing your work in a relaxed way or are tightening your jaw and neck – you must learn to relax. Just let yourself go loose and comfortable in your chair and think about relaxing your muscles, slow down your breathing and just BE.

'Let nothing disturb thee
Nothing affright thee
All things are passing
God never changeth'
ST TERESA OF AVILA

A few gentle stretches before bed, as in Lesson Six, will really help you sleep, but do remember that you must feed your soul as well as feeding your body. Before you turn off the light, try to read something inspirational and think about the positive things that have happened in your day. It is a good idea to keep a notebook of all the good things that happen to you each day, so that you can really see how much you have to be grateful for.

Creative Visualisation

When you are worrying about a difficult meeting or an important interview – or indeed any of life's traumas – lie down and relax each muscle in turn. Then, when your body is in a comfortable, drowsy state, visualise the outcome you desire. For example, imagine that important meeting you are concerned about and visualise it going perfectly. Visualise the people being receptive to your proposals and visualise a perfect outcome. Keep all this in your mind and plant it there. Take time to do this before every difficult occasion and it works! It is also much better for you than lying awake worrying.

Pregnancy

Yoga can be beneficial during pregnancy. If you have been practicing Yoga regularly prior to becoming pregnant, and have no history of miscarriage, have your doctor's consent and the guidance of a qualified teacher, there is no reason why you should not continue to practice. You must, of course, avoid all exercise that puts pressure on the abdomen – the Cobra, the Locust, the Bow, Salute to the Sun, the Pose of a Dog, the Pose of a Boat and the Abdominal Contractions and

Lift are all forbidden. As the abdomen gets larger, your teacher will aid you in adapting the positions to cope with your increasing size. But remember, you must advise your teacher if your blood pressure goes up.

Yoga breathing and the relaxation techniques will help you tremendously. The Cat Stretch (Lesson Four, pp56 -7) is excellent for relieving tension in the lower back, and the Thigh Stretch (Lesson Five, see p79) is really good for toning and stretching the inner thighs and keeping the hip joints flexible.

If you have never practiced Yoga before and would like to start Yoga in pregnancy, then it is best to wait until the fifteenth week. Make sure you have a good teacher and your doctor's permission.

'Anyone who actively practices yoga, be he young, old, or even very old, sickly or weak, can become a siddha [can acquire power].

Anyone who practices can acquire siddhis, but not he who is lazy. Yoga siddhis are not obtained by merely reading text-books.

Nor are they reached by wearing yoga garments or by conversation about yoga, but only through tireless practice. This is the secret of success. There is no doubt about it.'

HATHA YOGA PRADIPIKA (64-66)

BEFORE YOU BEGIN

Please try to do these Lessons in the order in which they are given because they have been tried and tested over the years and are arranged in a particular order to help you progress gradually and with care.

Yoga Breathing

A note on breathing. In these Lessons, all breathing is done through the nose, except where otherwise indicated. Yoga breathing will help the body and mind relax and as we breathe in deeply with every exercise we are encouraging richly oxygenated blood to all the tissues, helping them to positive health. As we exhale, we aid the elimination of toxins and waste products.

All the main instructions are given with each movement. Where no instruction is given, just breathe normally, and where inhale is not followed by exhale, exhale normally when you are ready.

To Practice Yoga

All you need is a warm, airy room, loose clothing and a rug, blanket or towel to sit on. Always leave about two hours after a meal before you start to practice. Practice without any strain at all and very quickly you will see the results.

Your body will become toned, your energy will improve and your stiffness will start to vanish.

The Golden Rule is *Never Ever Strain*. Just move slowly, carefully and gently into each movement, listening to your body and moving only at your own pace. Don't worry how stiff you are in the beginning, we all are – but that is why we do Yoga – and gradually as you keep practicing, your flexibility will improve tremendously. Even if you can only do a tiny bit of each movement to start with, just persevere and do remember that you will benefit at each stage of the movement.

Caution

Yoga is very beneficial for health but must never be used instead of your doctor's treatment. If you have any concerns whatsoever about the suitability of a particular exercise for you, please check with your doctor before you begin.

Now let's begin! I hope you enjoy the following Lessons. Please note that all the counts given are in seconds – but if you find them a little too much in the beginning, just halve them to start with.

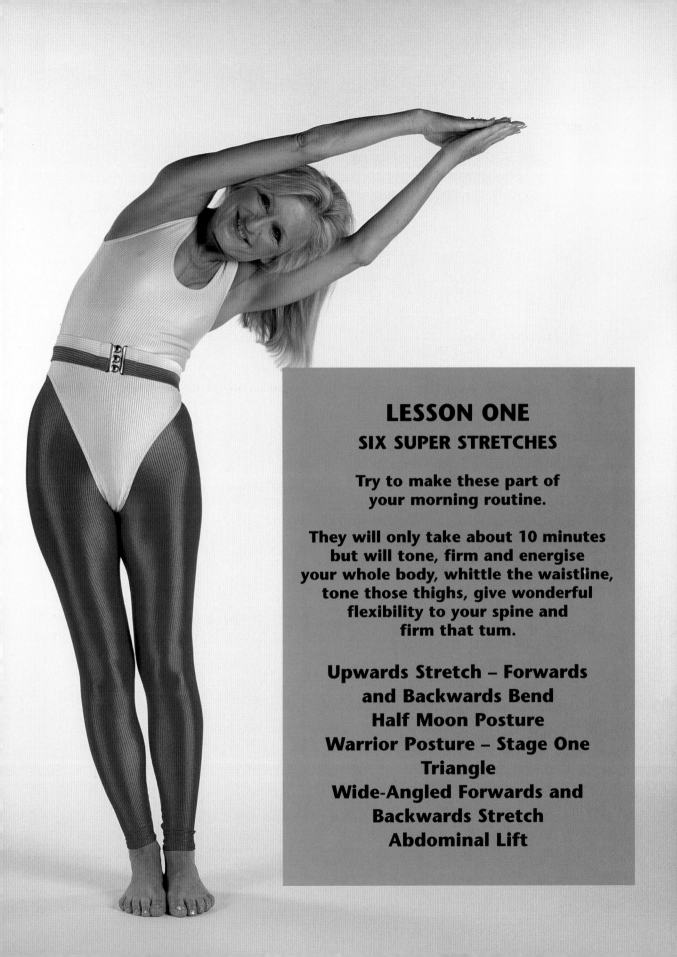

LESSON ONE
SIX SUPER STRETCHES

Try to make these part of
your morning routine.

They will only take about 10 minutes
but will tone, firm and energise
your whole body, whittle the waistline,
tone those thighs, give wonderful
flexibility to your spine and
firm that tum.

**Upwards Stretch – Forwards
and Backwards Bend
Half Moon Posture
Warrior Posture – Stage One
Triangle
Wide-Angled Forwards and
Backwards Stretch
Abdominal Lift**

UPWARDS STRETCH – FORWARDS AND BACKWARDS BEND

This is a marvellous movement to do first thing in the morning. It releases tension from the whole body, gently stretches and tones the spine, tones the muscles of the legs, firming the back of the thigh area, and is marvellous for the skin and hair due to the extra blood stimulated to the head and neck area.

● Stand very straight with your feet a little apart. Breathe in and slowly lift your arms, stretching them above your head.

Beginner's Hint

At first, the backwards bend part of this movement can be really difficult. To help prevent a fear of falling keep your arms straight, relax your neck and keep your eyes on your thumbs. Don't expect to move more than a couple of inches backwards in the beginning. Just keep practicing and you will be thrilled at how quickly you progress and how quickly your back acquires flexibility.

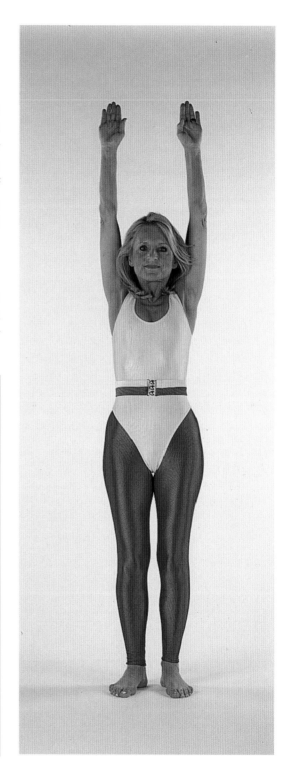

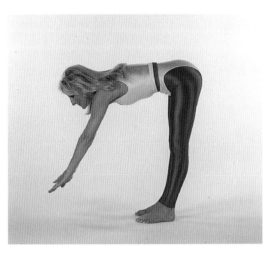

● Breathe out as you slowly and gently bend forwards, with your back flat and your head up, eventually reaching your maximum position *without strain*. Ensure your legs are straight. (Don't worry if you can only move a little to start with and your hands are nearer to your knees than your feet – just keep practicing and you'll soon be delighted with your progress.)

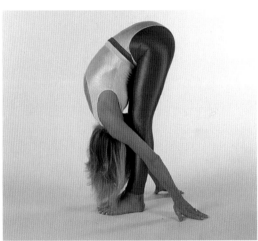

● Relax in your maximum position for a count of 5 seconds, breathing normally. The eventual aim is to have your chin between your knees – don't worry it will happen!

Now lift just the head and, breathing in, continue to lift your upper body until you are standing straight. Stretch your hands up above your head.

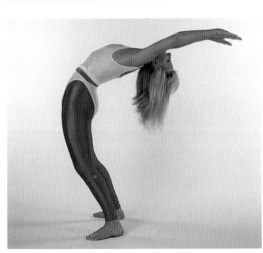

● With a full lung, gently stretch backwards exhaling in your maximum stretch. Breathe in and return to a standing position. Slowly lower your arms and relax. Repeat twice. As you progress, gradually increase the holds in this movement to 10 seconds, breathing normally in the maximum positions.

HALF MOON POSTURE

This brilliant exercise corrects posture, whittles the waistline, firms the back of the thighs and is excellent for the flexibility of the spine.

● Stand straight with your feet together. Inhale and lift your arms above your head, placing your hands together and crossing your thumbs. Make sure that the insides of your arms are beside your ears. Stretch upwards. Exhale as you slowly move your upper body to the right pushing the hips to the left, keeping your body in line, without moving forwards or backwards. Hold for 5 seconds. Inhale as you slowly return to an upright position and stretch up.

● Exhale as you move slowly to the left pushing your hips to the right. Hold for 5 seconds. Inhale as you slowly return to an upright position.

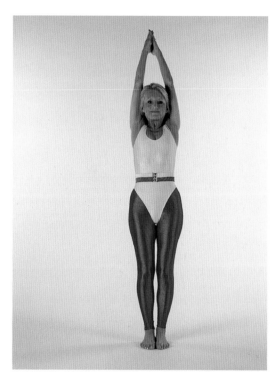

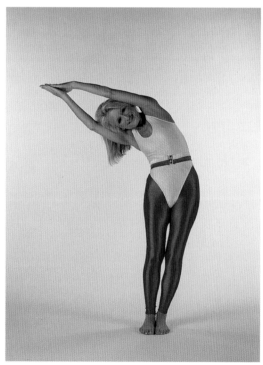

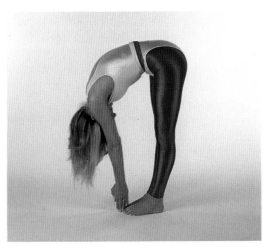

● Exhale as you move slowly forwards into your maximum forwards stretch. Hold for 5 seconds breathing normally. (Again, you probably won't be anywhere near the floor to start with. Just relax in yor maximum position even if it is only half way.)

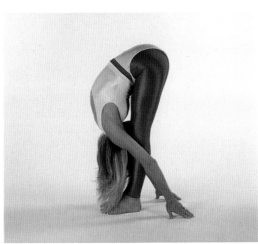

● Eventually you should aim to have your chin on your knees with your hands on the floor behind your feet. Don't strain, all it takes is perseverance. Inhale as you slowly return to an upright position.

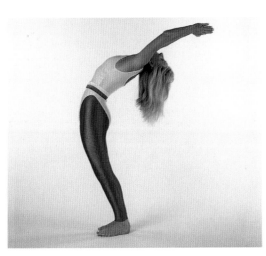

● Now stretch back with a full lung exhaling in your maximum position (don't worry if you are only stretching back a couple of inches at first). Inhale as you return to an upright position. Exhale, lower your arms and relax. Repeat once.

WARRIOR POSTURE

Stage One

This movement is magnificent for firming the thighs, buttocks and calves. It is excellent for helping to remove cellulite and maintaining the flexibility of the hips.

● Stand straight with your legs about 3-4 feet apart. Place your right foot so it faces to the right side and have your left foot pointing forwards. Inhale and lift your arms out at the sides.

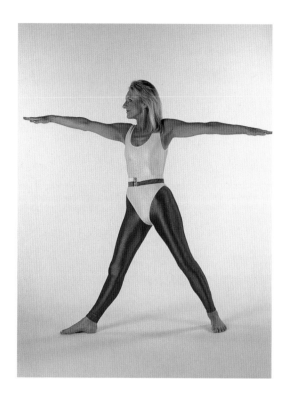

● Exhale and, keeping your body straight, bend your right knee aiming eventually to have your thigh totally flat and your left leg straight. Make sure your left foot stays flat on the floor. Hold for a count of 5, breathing normally. Inhale and return to an upright position. Repeat to the left side.

Beginner's Hint
Keeping your thigh flat may seem impossible at first. Don't worry, keep trying, remember you don't have to manage the perfect position to benefit – your best is all you need to do. Soon you will be rewarded by slimmer, toned thighs!

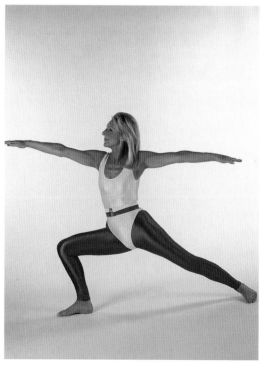

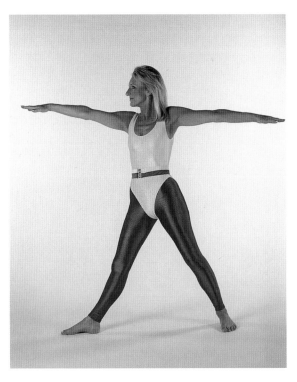

TRIANGLE

This movement is great for hips, ankles, knees and thighs and is brilliant for keeping the flexibility in the lower back. It also reduces flab around the waist and hips and stimulates blood flow to all the spinal nerves.

● Stand straight with your legs about 4 feet apart. Place your right foot at 90 degrees to the right and have your left foot facing forwards. Inhale and lift your arms straight out at the sides.

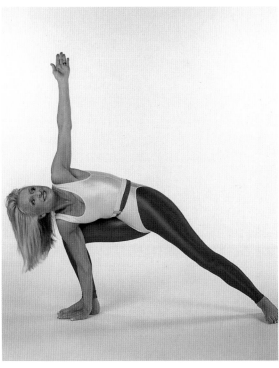

● As you exhale bend your right knee and clasp your right foot with your right hand. If you can't reach just hold your leg wherever is comfortable. (If possible place your hand flat on the floor, with little finger by big toe.) Lift your left arm up and turn your head to look at the ceiling, pulling your shoulder back so that your finger- tips point to the ceiling. Hold for 5, inhale and return to a standing position. Repeat on the other side, then repeat the exercise.

WIDE–ANGLED FORWARDS AND BACKWARDS STRETCH

This movement is excellent for toning and firming the backs of the legs and buttocks. It's a wonderful stretch for those who work at a desk all day long, it relieves tightness in the chest and gives the spine amazing flexibility and has proved helpful to asthma sufferers.

● Stand with your legs about 3 feet apart and stretch upwards as you inhale.

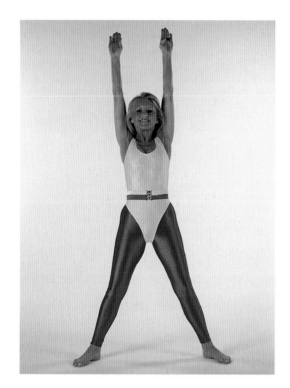

● Exhale and, keeping your head up, your back flat and your legs straight, allow your body to move carefully forwards.

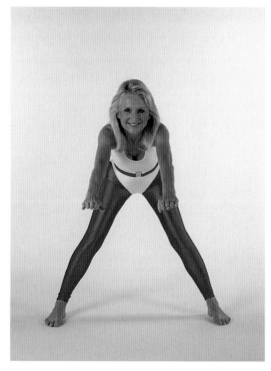

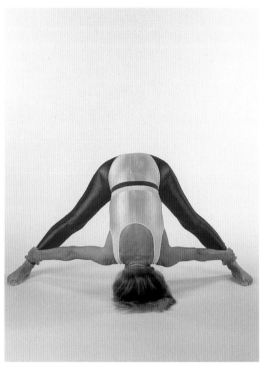

● On reaching your maximum position without strain, clasp your legs wherever you can reach and draw your head in towards your knees. Eventually you will be able to clasp your ankles and bring your head to the floor, but *please* don't strain.

Beginner's Hint

At first the head and the floor seem miles apart but by literally hanging in there and allowing gravity to help, your back will acquire a flexibility you never thought possible.

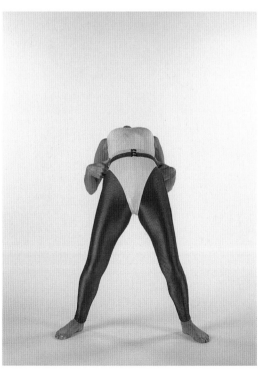

● Lift just your head, then start to inhale as you gently come up into a standing position. Gently stretch the body upwards then, with a full lung, place your thumbs in front of your waistline and fingers towards your back and gently relax your body backwards. Exhale and hold for a count of 5, breathing normally. Inhale as you return to a standing position. Exhale, relax and repeat.

ABDOMINAL LIFT

**CAUTION:
DO NOT ATTEMPT IF YOU
ARE PREGNANT**

**These movements must be done
on an empty stomach.**

Your abdomen drops as you get older, so the abdominal lift is invaluable for keeping the abdomen firm, uplifted and youthful. When you first start this movement, the abdomen might not move very much. Just persevere and soon you'll be delighted with the results – a firmer, flatter tum.

● Stand straight and take a deep breath, bend slightly forwards, exhale fully and, keeping the air out of the lungs, pull the abdomen in and up and hold for a count of 10. Relax, inhale and repeat 3 times.

ABDOMINAL CONTRACTIONS

This movement stimulates peristalsis and helps relieve constipation.

● Standing straight, inhale deeply then, bending slightly forwards, exhale fully and, keeping the air out of the lungs, snap the abdomen in and out 10 times, gradually increasing to 20 times with practice.

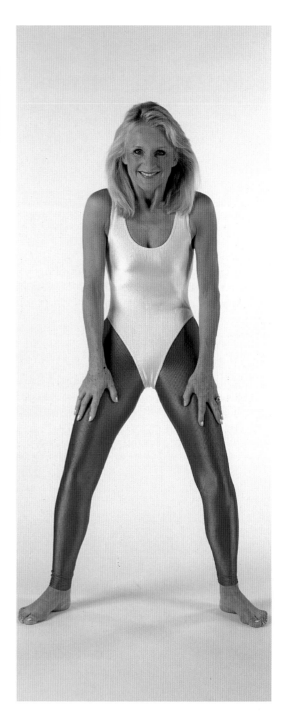

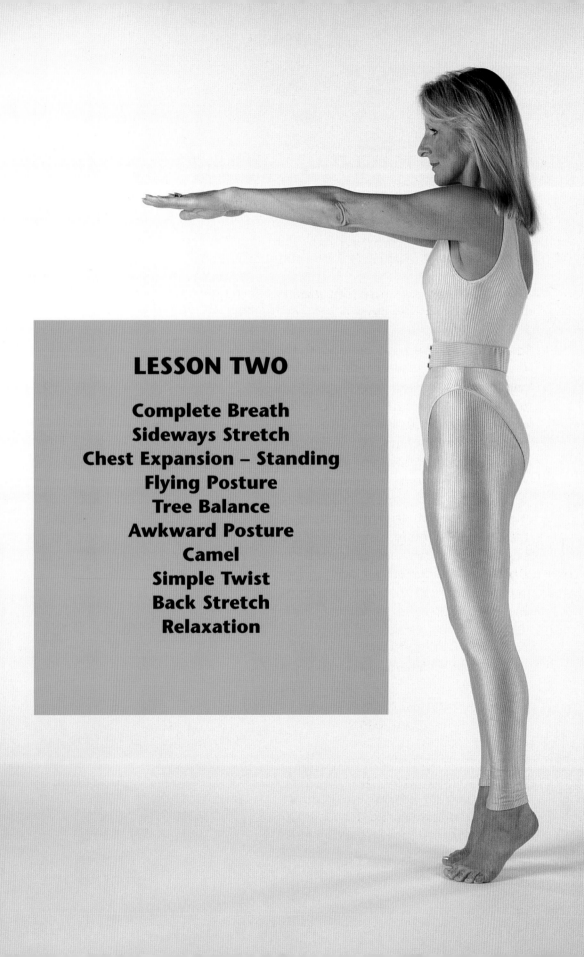

LESSON TWO

Complete Breath
Sideways Stretch
Chest Expansion – Standing
Flying Posture
Tree Balance
Awkward Posture
Camel
Simple Twist
Back Stretch
Relaxation

COMPLETE BREATH

A Yoga saying is 'Life is breath and he who only half breathes, only half lives'. It is very sad that today most people only use about one third of their lung capacity. They would have much more energy and feel much more relaxed if their lungs were used properly.

The complete breath uses all the lung capacity. We push the abdominal muscles out as we breathe in. The diaphragm then drops and the bottom of the lung inflates. We then continue to breathe in to inflate the whole lungs, retaining the air and increasing the possibility of more oxygen absorption. At the end of the slow exhalation we pull the abdominal muscles in and up to push the stale air from the bottom of the lungs. We push the abdominal muscles out and breathe in again.

Slow, deep breathing will always help you relax. You do not have to do the arm movement when you have learned this exercise, so why not learn to slow down your breathing wherever you are – on the bus, at work, wherever – especially when stressed. It will make you feel so much better and look so much younger, relax your whole body and focus and sharpen your mind.

● Stand very straight with your hands by your sides and your feet about 1 foot apart. Push your abdominal muscles out and start to breathe in – keep breathing in through your nose and slowly raise your arms above your head. Hold your breath for a count of 5 and then slowly breathe out through the nose; take 5 seconds to do this, lowering your arms to your sides.

● At the end of your exhalation, pull your abdominal muscles in and up, push them out and start breathing in. Repeat 10 times.

● As you practice you will find your breathing capacity expands so gradually increase your inhalations and exhalations at your own pace. But *never* strain the lungs. Eventually you will be able to inhale for 10 seconds, hold for 10 seconds and exhale for 10 seconds.

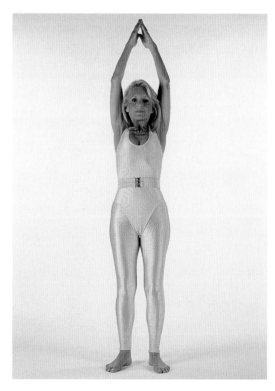

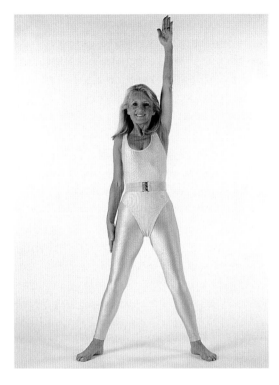

SIDEWAYS STRETCH

This movement keeps the small of the back area beautifully supple and is a wonderful movement for slimming and firming the midriff and waistline. There is no need for an expanding waistline or a flabby spare tyre. This movement will help keep them away for ever.

● Stand straight with your legs about three feet apart and your hands by your side. Breathe in and lift your left hand in the air.

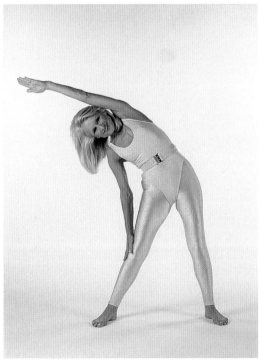

● Stretch this arm up, then, breathing out and bending to the right side, slowly slide your right hand down your right leg. Do not strain, and hold your maximum position for a count of 5, increasing to 10 as your confidence in the movement increases. Breathe in and slowly return to a standing position. Repeat to the other side and relax. Repeat the entire movement twice on each side.

CHEST EXPANSION – STANDING

This is a lovely stretch to start your day, but is also a wonderful movement to help release tension in the neck and shoulder area. So many people suffer from pains and stiffness in the neck, either physical pain due to overwork, or mentally induced through tension and stress. Nothing is more damaging to the way you look than a tense expression and, if allowed to continue, this condition frequently gives rise to headaches and a feeling of extreme tiredness. This exercise relaxes the shoulder and neck area, and by so doing, allows the circulation to flow freely to the head and neck, so benefiting your skin, hair and brain cells. It also stretches the spine and tones the muscles of the legs, firms the bust, tones the upper arm area and improves posture.

● Stand very straight with your feet together and interlock your fingers behind your back.

● Breathe in and, slowly breathing out, bend forwards lifting your arms up as high as possible. Relax in your maximum forwards bend for a count of 5, breathing normally.

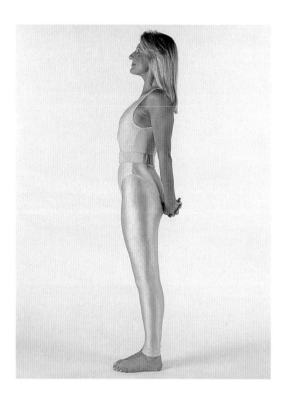

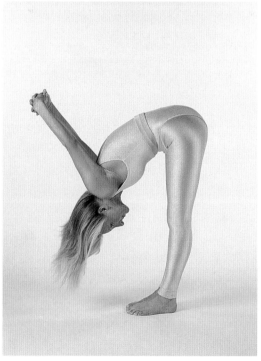

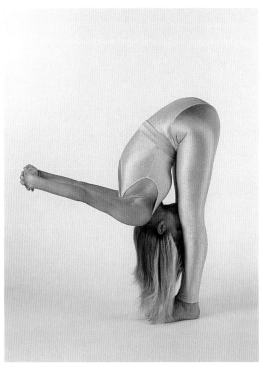

● With practice your chin will reach your knees and your arms will lift a little higher. But do remember this will come – don't strain.

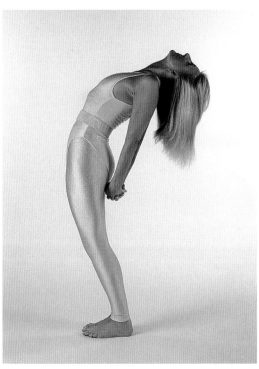

● Breathe in and slowly lift your head, coming up into an upright position. With a full lung bend backwards, pulling your hands down under your bottom, exhale and hold for a count of 5, breathing normally. Breathe in and slowly come up into an upright position. Breathe out, lower your arms and relax. Repeat 3 times.

FLYING POSTURE

The balances in Yoga help to give a feeling of poise and confidence. They are also very important for sharpening the powers of concentration and balance – in fact I have been told by many of my golf and tennis playing students that these balancing postures have helped their game tremendously! This movement tones the muscles of the upper arm area, the chest and the legs, keeps the hips flexible and helps prevent the bottom from dropping.

● Stand straight and take your left foot behind your right foot, your fingertips touching at chest level.

'The mind in
its own place and
in itself can make
a Heaven of Hell
and a Hell of Heaven.'

JOHN MILTON
(1608-1674)

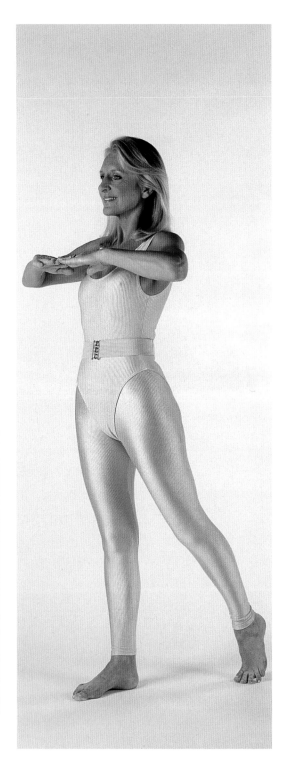

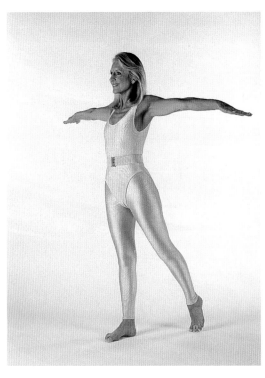

● Breathe in deeply and spread your arms out at shoulder level, then exhale.

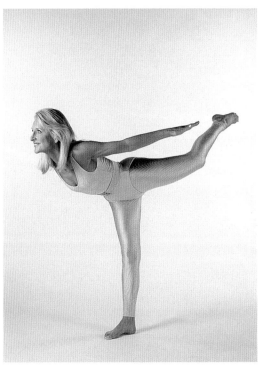

● Breathe in again and as you exhale, slowly lift your left leg as high as you can behind you, at the same time lower your upper body slightly. Hold your maximum position for a count of 5, concentrating on a spot to help you balance, and then slowly come back to an upright position. Place your hands together, stand straight and relax. Repeat on the other side. Then repeat the movement once on each side. Gradually increase the hold to 10 as you become confident in the movement.

TREE BALANCE

This exercise tones and firms the muscles of the inner and outer thighs. It helps to keep the hips, knees and ankles really flexible. But, as with all yoga exercises, the secret is to persevere *without strain* – you are doing very well and will get there, don't overdo it!

● Stand straight and place your left foot on your right thigh. (When you first try to do this it is quite difficult, as the aim is to place the foot as shown in the picture below, but the foot can be placed on the inner thigh, the calf or the knee – or even the ankle in the beginning – until your joints are sufficiently flexible to enable you to do this.)

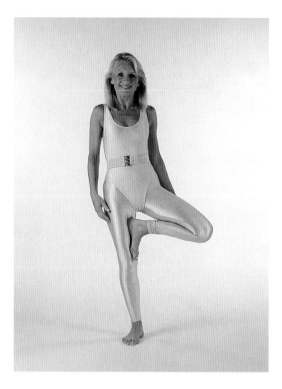

● Breathe in, lift your arms above your head and with your palms together, stretch up. Hold for a count of 5, breathing normally. Keep your eyes focused on a spot to help your concentration. This is the secret that helps you to balance. Slowly lower your arms and your leg and repeat on the other side. Then repeat on both sides, gradually increasing the hold to 10 as you gain confidence.

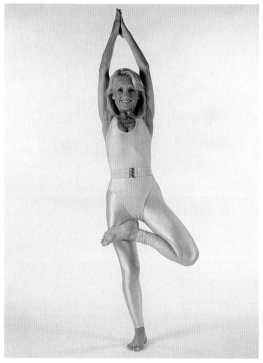

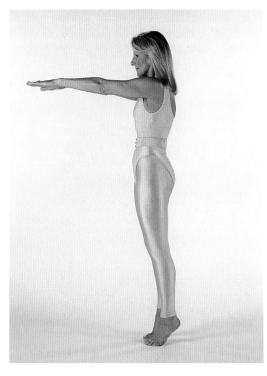

AWKWARD POSTURE

This brilliant movement tones and firms the front of the thighs, improves the flexibility of the knees and strengthens the arches, toes and ankles.

● Stand straight, with your feet about 1 foot apart, hands parallel to the floor and rise up on to your toes.

● Take a deep breath, exhale and gently lower your bottom as far as possible to your heels, keeping your back straight. Don't worry if at first you can only go half way. This is quite normal. Slowly breathe in and return to an upright position. Repeat 3 times.

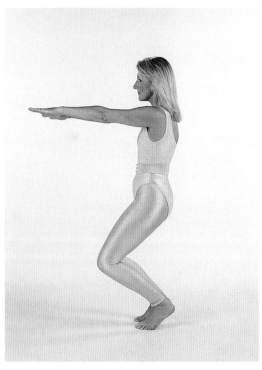

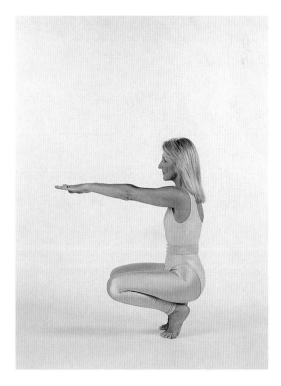

CAMEL

This exercise improves the jawline, firms the abdomen and slims the midriff and the waistline. It removes tightness from the neck and shoulders, it expands the rib cage and promotes slow, deep relaxed breathing. Because 90 per cent of our normal daily movements are forwards, it is easy to develop poor posture and the dreaded stoop. This brilliant movement is the answer! If you find it difficult at first, just keep practicing and gradually you will be able to do it, but *never* move further than your own maximum position.

● Adopt a high kneeling position with your hands at your waistline, thumbs in front and fingers behind supporting the lower back, knees and feet one foot apart.

● Breathe in deeply, and allow your upper body to bend backwards, keeping your thighs straight. Exhale once you have reached your maximum position.

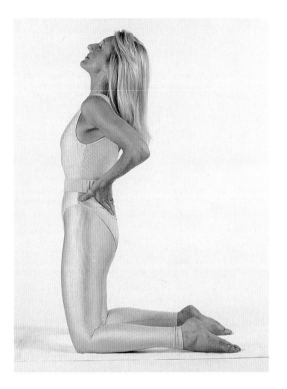

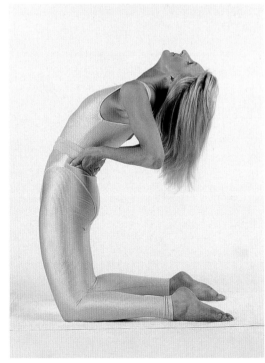

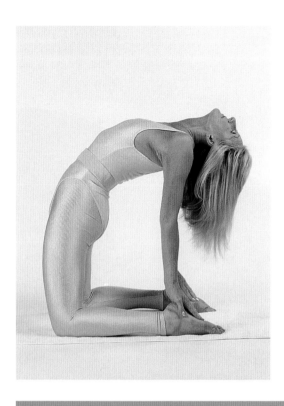

● If you can, place your right hand on your right foot and your left hand on your left foot. If you can't, just keep your hands at your waistline and hold your maximum position, breathing normally, for a count of 5. (As your flexibility improves, gradually increase the hold to a count of 10.) Inhale as you return to an upright position.

● Exhale and allow your bottom to sink to your heels, with your hands by your sides and your head on the floor. This unwinds your spine and is called the Pose of a Child. Hold this position for a count of 5, breathing normally. Then inhale and return to an upright position and repeat the entire movement.

Life has reached such a hectic pace that it is not surprising that more people are suffering from stress. We are walking around with muscles in an uptight state, as though they are literally squeezed together, so consequently we feel squeezed, both mentally and physically.

More and more people are taking pills to help them relax, pills to help them sleep, pills to relieve headaches and alcohol to help them unwind - but is this really the answer?

Once you start practicing Yoga you will realise that the brilliant stretches go systematically around your whole body, relieving tensions that might have been lingering for ages.

SIMPLE TWIST

This marvellous exercise helps to relieve tension from the spine, aiding the flexibility of both back and neck. It helps slim the thighs and waistline and carefully massages the abdominal organs.

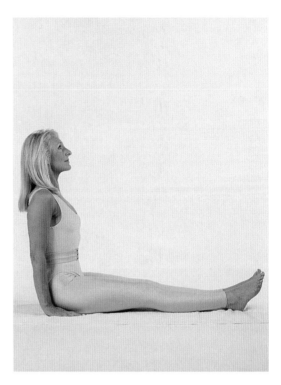

● Sit with your legs straight out in front you. Take a deep breath in and lift your right foot over your left thigh, place your right hand on the floor behind your back.

● Gently stretch your left hand over on the outside of your right knee and place it on your left knee. If you can't reach to begin with just do your best.

● Gently turn your head over your right shoulder and gradually twist the whole torso to the right. Hold for a count of 5. Slowly return your head to the front and repeat on the other side. Then repeat the entire movement.

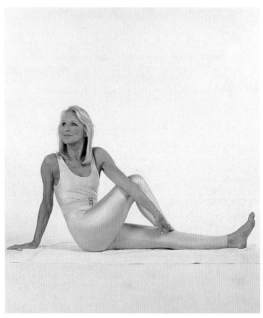

BACK STRETCH

The Yoga saying 'You are as young as your spine is flexible' rings so true – you have only to watch a crowd to see how a stiff back ages people. Don't worry if your lower back is stiff and your hamstrings are really tight to start with. Most people start like this but very quickly you will acquire flexibility and feel revitalised. With this movement you can improve the flexibility of the spine and firm the abdominal area and the back of the legs.

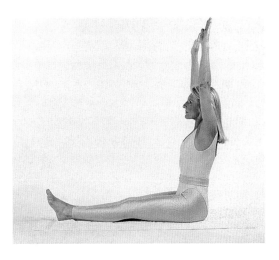

● With both legs straight out in front of you, breathe in and slowly stretch your arms up as high as possible. Exhale and stretch forwards without strain.

● Clasp your legs and gently lower your chin to your knees keeping your head up until the last moment.

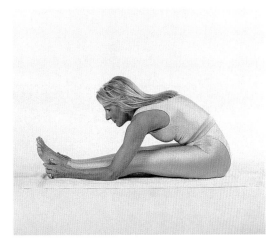

● Eventually with practice you will be able to clasp your feet – or even stretch your hands past your feet – and lower your chin to your knees but don't strain. Relax and hold your maximum position for a count of 5, increasing the hold gradually to 10 as your flexibility improves. Breathe in and return to your seated position. Repeat 3 times.

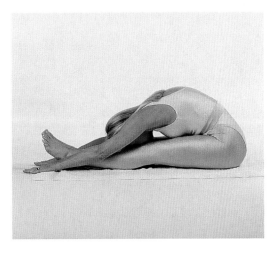

RELAXATION

● Lie flat on your back and gently lift your knees up to your chest. Interlock you hands together around your knees, and gently rock from one side to the other. Let your legs go straight out in front of you and your arms fall to the floor and relax.

● Lie flat, with your legs apart and your arms about one foot from your body, palms facing upwards. Just allow your body to go completely limp and heavy. Put all thoughts out of your mind. Keep your breathing slow and deep and then, starting with your feet, concentrate on relaxing each muscle in turn, until you have relaxed every muscle in your body. Close your eyes and let your eyelids go very heavy. Let your eyeballs roll upwards and your scalp slide back. Feel yourself relaxing more and more.

● Now imagine that you are very warm on a beautiful beach – imagine the waves are gently lapping on the shore – every time you breathe in try to imagine the waves coming slowly towards you and every time you breathe out imagine them going slowly back into the sea again. Relax for 5 or 10 minutes. After you have fully relaxed, take a deep breath, have a beautiful stretch and make the most of your day.

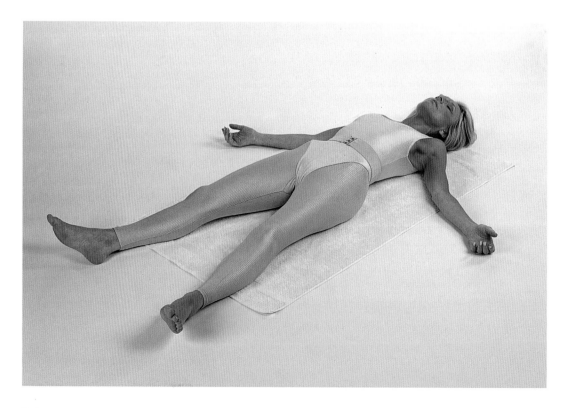

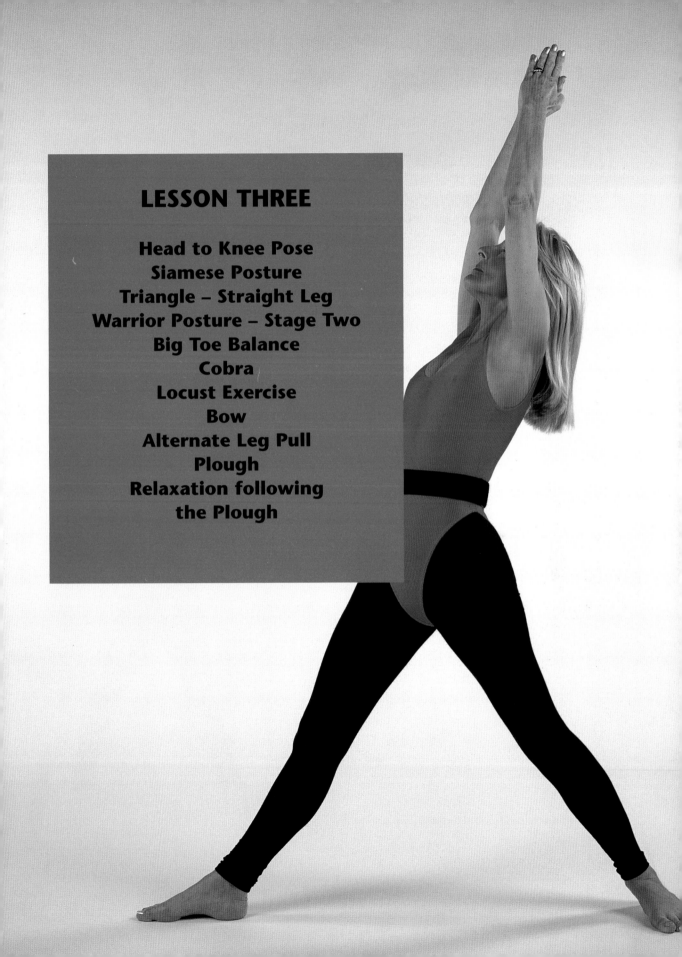

LESSON THREE

HEAD TO KNEE POSE

This movement tones the backs of the thighs and calves promotes great spinal flexibility. Remember when you first start, it is usual to find one side is easier than the other. Yoga will gradually help straighten out your imbalances.

● Stand straight, placing your left foot 3 feet in front of your right. Inhale, and place both arms straight above your head, palms together, thumbs crossed.

Yoga has helped me maintain good posture and keep supple. It has also helped to keep my stomach flat and to tone up my thighs. No matter how tired I feel at the beginning of the class, I always feel energised by the end.

G.B.

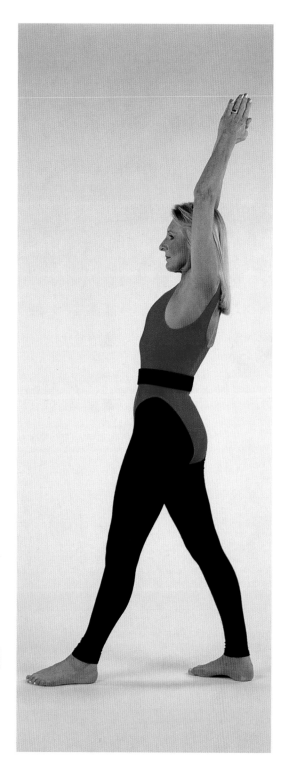

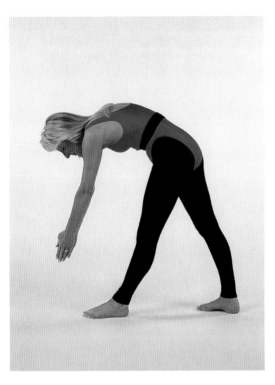

● Exhale and bend forwards, aiming to clasp your left foot and put your chin on your left knee. This is rarely possible to begin with. Just do your best, but notice how far away your head is from your knee on this side. Inhale and return to a standing posture. Repeat to the other side. Again, go carefully, and notice the distance between your chin and knee.

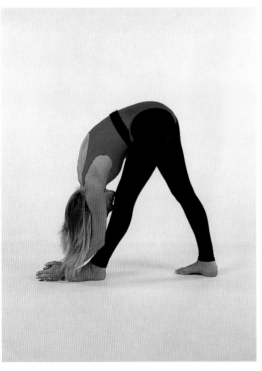

● As you progress in the movement, you will eventually be able to clasp your foot and place your chin on your knee on both sides – but don't strain. Inhale, lift the head and the arms and stretch up. Then relax and repeat the movement.

SIAMESE POSTURE

This movement gives extra firmness to the midriff and waistline and is excellent for keeping the spine flexible.

● Stand straight with your feet about 3 feet apart. Place your right hand on top of your head and look into the elbow.

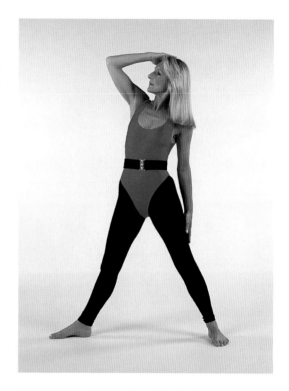

● Inhale deeply and as you exhale gently slide your left hand down your left leg. Hold for a count of 5, then inhale and return to a standing position. Repeat on the other side and then repeat on each side.

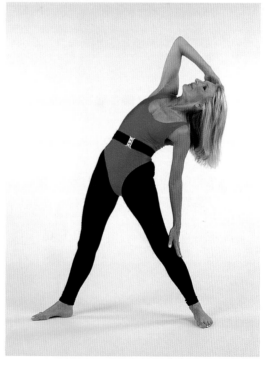

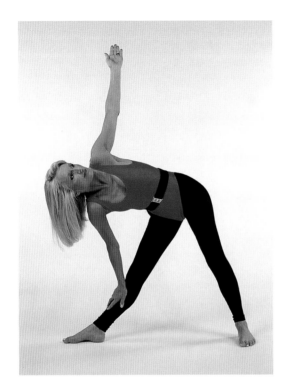

TRIANGLE – STRAIGHT LEG

We did the Triangle in Lesson One (see p17) but now let's try it with straight legs. Again, this great exercise keeps the lower back agile. This shows in the way you walk and get up out of a chair. It is also super for the flexibility of your hips and is excellent for toning the backs of the thighs and the spinal nerves and reducing flab around the waist and hips.

● Stand straight and place your legs about 4 feet apart with your right foot at 90 degrees, your left foot facing forwards and your arms out at the sides. Inhale, and as you exhale keep your right leg straight and, gently bending to your right, clasp it with your right hand.

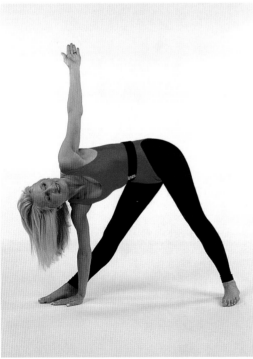

● If possible, place your hand flat on the floor with little finger by big toe. Lift your left arm up straight and turn your head to look at the ceiling, pulling your shoulder back so your fingertips point to the ceiling. Hold for a count of 5, increasing to 10 as your confidence builds, inhale and return to a standing position. Repeat on the other side Repeat the exercise.

WARRIOR POSTURE

Stage Two

In Lesson 1, (see p16) we did the Warrior Posture Stage One. Here is a slightly stronger version that helps prevent stiffness in the lower back and hips. It is brilliant for removing flab from the hips and removes stiffness and tension from the shoulders. It also helps you acquire lovely lean thighs and legs.

● Stand straight with your feet about 4 feet apart, your right foot at 90 degrees and your left foot facing front. Place your hands above your head, palms together, arms straight, and point the fingers to the ceiling, crossing your thumbs.

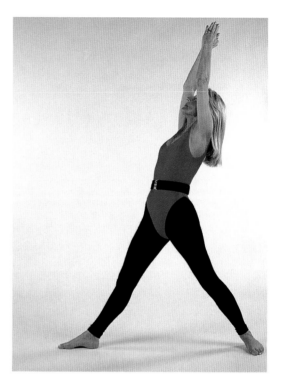

● Inhale and as you exhale bend the right knee aiming to flatten your thigh so that it is parallel to the floor (don't worry, this takes a while – *don't strain*). Drop your head back, look at your hands and, breathing normally, stay in the pose for a count of 5. Inhale slowly and return to an upright position. Repeat on the other side. Then repeat the whole sequence.

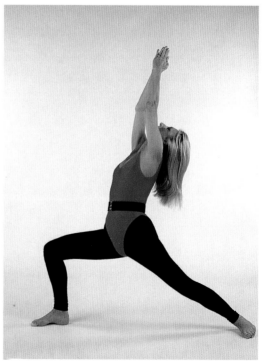

BIG TOE BALANCE

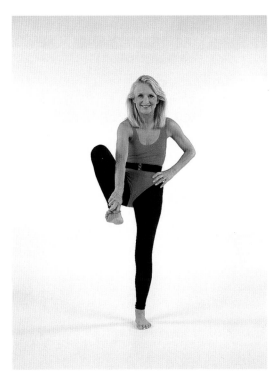

The benefits of this balance include lifting the bottom and firming the backs of the thighs. You can almost feel the cellulite being removed! The hips stay really flexible and, as with all balances, it really helps you clear your mind as well as improving your concentration.

● Stand straight and place your left hand on your left hip. Breathe in and clasp your right big toe in your right hand.

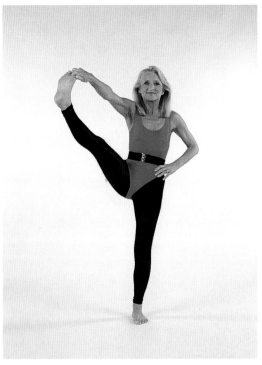

● As you exhale (concentrate on a spot to help you balance) gradually stretch out your right leg. Don't worry if it isn't straight to begin with – just practice and it soon will be. Hold for a count of 5, then lower and repeat to the other side. As your confidence in the position increases gradually increase the hold to a count of 10. Repeat once on each side.

41

COBRA

**CAUTION:
DO NOT ATTEMPT IF YOU
ARE PREGNANT**

This is a very beautiful backwards stretch – it tones and firms the muscles in the chin and jaw, it removes tension from the shoulder area, tones the upper arms, firms the buttocks, corrects poor posture, tones the bust, helps remove toxins from the body and is also excellent for helping to relieve menstrual problems like cramps and lower back ache.

● Lie on your stomach with your legs together, your chin on the floor and your hands either side, just below shoulder level and three inches from your body. Breathe in and slowly lift your head and shoulders off the floor. Keep the lower abdomen on the floor. Do not strain.

● Keep lifting until you reach your maximum position. Often, the halfway stage is all one can reach to begin with.

● As you progress, let your head drop back to look at the ceiling, exhale and hold this position, breathing normally, for a count of 5. Slowly lower your body to the floor, place your forehead on the floor, then turn your head to one side and relax.

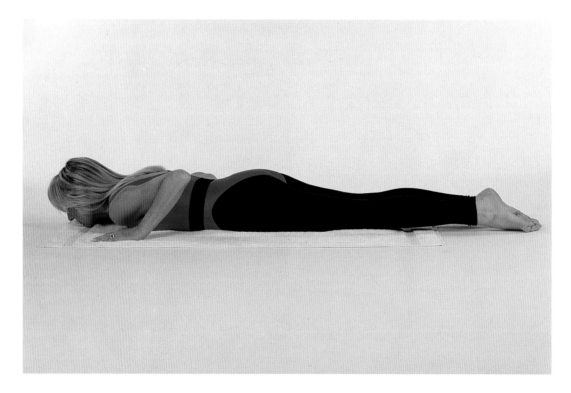

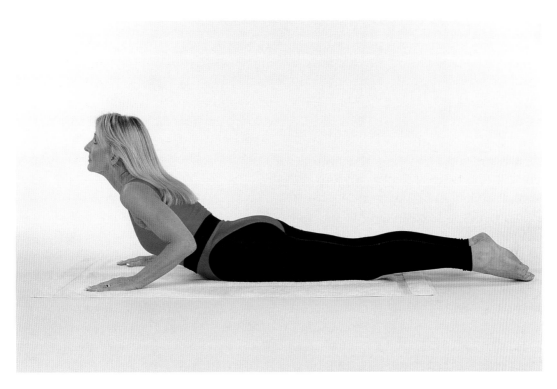

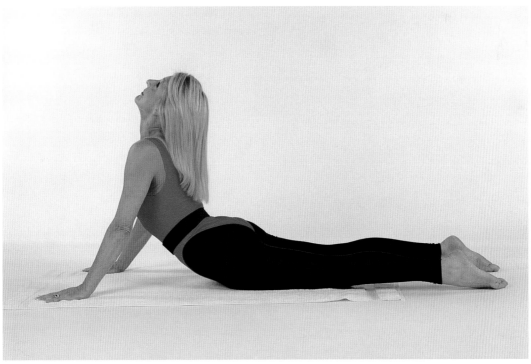

LOCUST EXERCISE

**CAUTION:
DO NOT ATTEMPT IF YOU
ARE PREGNANT**

This is brilliant for lifting the bottom, firming the backs of the thighs and strengthening the lower back. Weak lower backs are common as we get older. The Locust adds strength in this area, thus preventing problems, it also helps prevent the dreaded sagging bottom. Sometimes before bed our minds are overactive and it is difficult to switch off. If you practice this posture before bed it can give you the help you need. You will not need a lullaby!

Half Locust

● Lie on your stomach, with your chin on the floor and your hands by your sides. Breathe in and then exhale and lift your left leg as high as possible, keeping it straight. Hold for a count of 5 then slowly lower it. Repeat on the other side, then repeat on both sides.

Full Locust

● Lying on your stomach, fold your fingers around your thumbs, and place both arms underneath your body, elbows as well.

● Breathe in and then exhale and lift both legs. Keep them a little apart at first. Eventually, as you practice the movement and feel more comfortable in it, try to keep the legs together and straight. Hold for a count of 3 to begin with and increase to 5 as you practice the movement. Repeat twice.

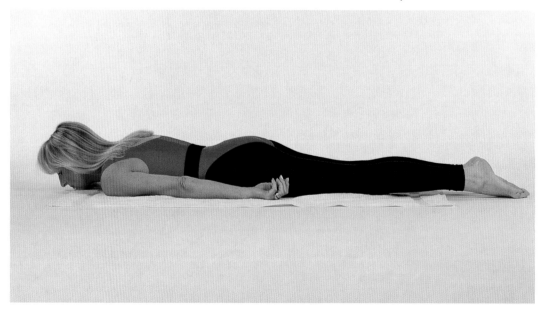

HALF LOCUST

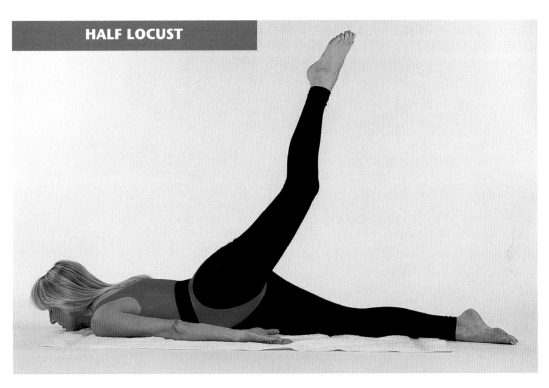

FULL LOCUST

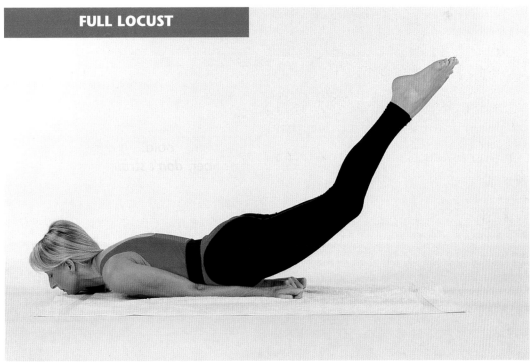

BOW

**CAUTION:
DO NOT ATTEMPT IF YOU
ARE PREGNANT**

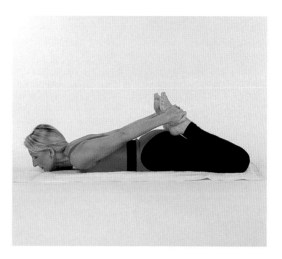

This is one of Yoga's best age defying movements. Start it today and practice it daily; it seems to melt all the tensions from your spine. It often proves quite difficult in the beginning but, again, do persevere; it's really worth it, as it helps remove stiffness from the neck and shoulders, massages all the internal organs, promotes flexibility in the spine, firms thighs and arms, and is a great help for women with menstrual problems.

● Lie on the floor face down with your chin on the floor. Inhale and clasp your feet in your hands with your hands on the outside of your feet. If you can't reach your feet at first don't worry, put your socks on, let the toes hang loose and hang on to the socks! Exhale and hold for a second.

● Now inhale and lift your head and feet to your maximum position without strain. Exhale and remain in the position for a count of 5, breathing normally. Then gently lower your body to the floor and relax and repeat once only.

● When and *only when* your body has become a little more supple, try rocking backwards and forwards in your

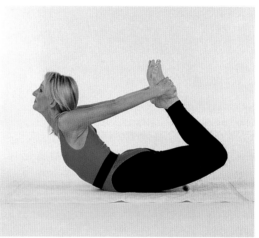

maximum hold. Gently does it, remember, *don't strain*!

● Following the bow, lie flat on your tum, then gently lift your bottom to your heels, place your forehead on the floor in front of your knees and relax in the Pose of a Child to refresh your spine.

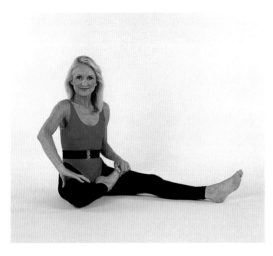

ALTERNATE LEG PULL

This movement loosens the hip joints and restores flexibility to the knees, feet and ankles. It gently stretches the spine and the muscles in the legs. When people start practicing this movement they are frequently amazed about how stiff their hips have become. But always remember, do not strain, keep practicing and very quickly your body will loosen up. This gentle movement will help keep your hips in excellent condition for life and put a spring back in your step!

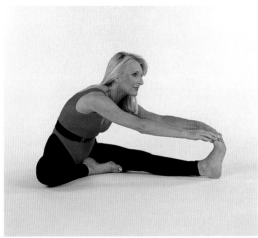

● Sitting straight, place your right foot on your left thigh, gently bouncing the flexed knee up and down to loosen the hip joint. If your foot is not comfortable on your upper thigh, just place it in the middle, between your legs. Now place both hands parallel to the outstretched leg and take a deep breath in. Lift the arms above the head, keeping them straight.

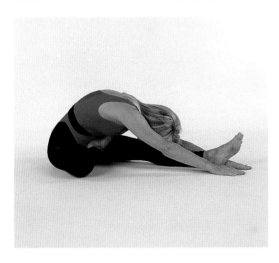

● Breathe out and very slowly stretch forwards aiming to clasp your left foot with both hands and gently take your head towards your knee. Relax in your maximum position for a count of 5, then slowly breathe in and return to a sitting position. Breathe out, relax and repeat to the other side. Perform this movement twice on each side.

PLOUGH

This is a wonderfully relaxing movement – it gently stretches and removes tension from the whole spine. It benefits the skin and hair, firms the buttocks and is a wonderful movement to do at the end of a busy day. The Yoga inverted positions stimulate blood to the skin and hair. Remember, our blood feeds our brain, skin and hair. The effects of these movements help you to a lovely radiant glow and also boosts your energy.

● Lie flat on your back with your hands relaxed by your sides. Breathe in, then breathe out and with bent knees slowly lift both your legs and buttocks off the floor. Lift them as far as you can without strain, supporting your back by placing your hands at your waistline. Then hold your maximum position as long as is comfortable (start at 10 seconds, and gradually increase to 30 seconds, as you practice you may wish to hold this movement for 3 minutes but increase it *gradually* at the rate of 30 seconds per week).

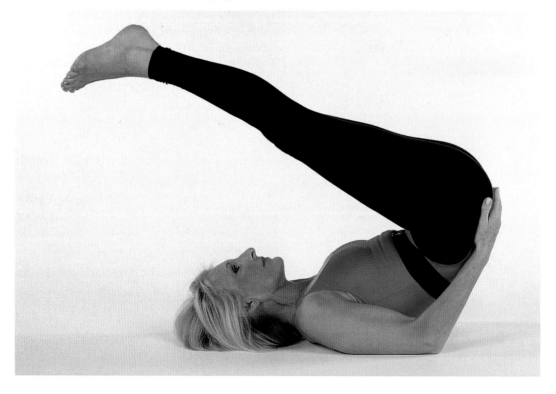

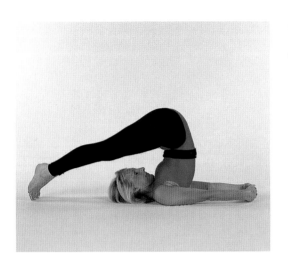

● As your spine becomes more supple your feet will touch the floor and your hands may be placed on the floor and interlocked together. Don't rush, just progress at your own pace.

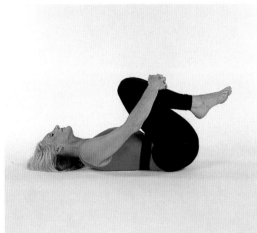

● To come out of this position, lower your knees to your forehead, and then gently roll, one vertebra at a time, down your back until your bottom touches the floor. Then slowly stretch both legs straight out in front of you and relax. Gently draw both knees to your chest and rock your back from side to side to relax the lower back and then let both legs go straight out in front of you and relax.

I have only recently taken up Yoga but am already reaping the benefits. Working in a high pressure job, it is sometimes hard to get a perspective on life and take 'time-out'. Yoga helps me to relax whilst toning me up at the same time!

N.P.

RELAXATION
FOLLOWING THE PLOUGH

Lie flat on your back. Make sure you are warm enough and consciously relax each muscle in turn. Let all the tension drain from your mind and body.

Slow your breathing down and now visualise a beautiful sunrise. See a golden sun slowly rising. Focus on the beautiful colours in the sky and see the sun glowing warm, golden and radiant,

giving light, warmth and energy.

Now visualise your own body bathed in early morning sunlight, and relax, relax, relax.

Relax for 5 to 10 minutes. Then slowly stretch and gently come up into a sitting position.

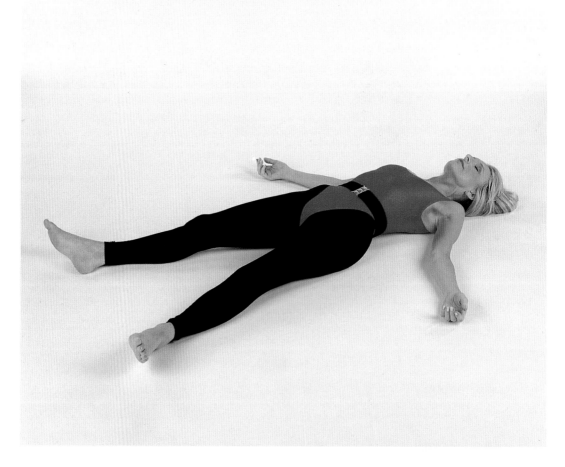

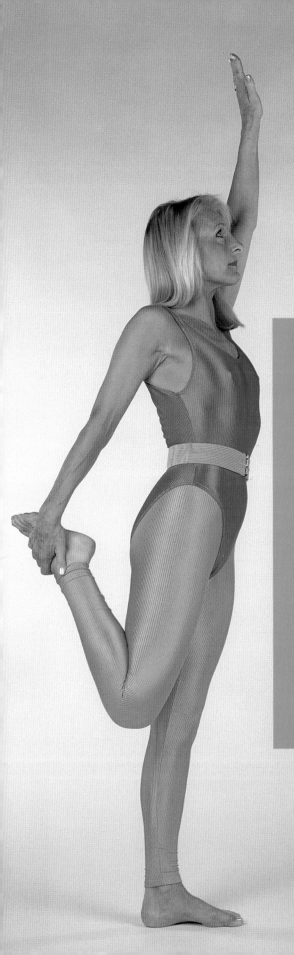

LESSON FOUR

RISHIS POSTURE

The Rishis Posture is excellent for removing lower back and shoulder stiffness. It tones and firms the backs of the calves and thighs.

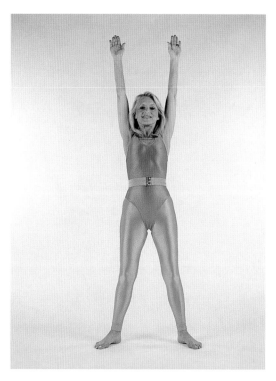

● Stand straight, with your feet about 2 feet apart. Breathe in and lift both arms in the air.

● Exhale and slowly bend forward to your own maximum position. Clasp your left leg with your right hand and slowly lift your left arm in the air, looking up at the palm of the hand. Do not strain, breathe normally in the position and hold for a count of 5.

● Gradually lower your left arm and relax in your maximum forwards bend. Then, inhaling, lift your head and gradually return to a standing position, stretch your arms above your head and, exhaling, lower them. Repeat on the other side. Then repeat the entire routine. As you practice this movement you will find that your flexibility improves so much that eventually you will be able to clasp your ankle.

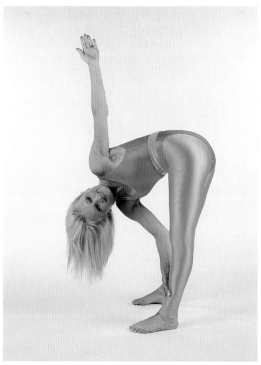

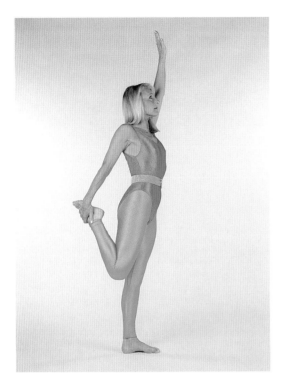

DANCER'S POSTURE

This beautiful movement is great for toning and firming the front of the thighs and for lifting the bottom. It also maintains great flexibility for the legs and shoulders and helps your concentration and balance.

● Stand straight and, placing your left hand straight up in the air, collect your right toes in your right hand, behind your back.

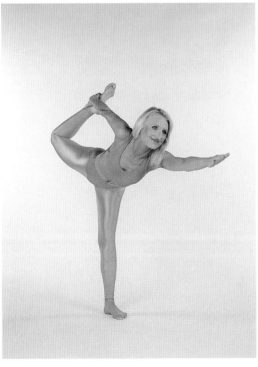

● Breathe in and as you exhale lift your right leg as high as possible while leaning forwards. Don't worry if it does not lift much to begin with – it will with practice. Hold for 5 at first, increasing gradually to a count of 10. Return to an upright position, lower your leg, place your hands together and relax. Then repeat on the other side and repeat the sequence on both sides.

EAGLE BALANCE

This is a wonderful movement to encourage flexibility in the shoulders, arms, elbows, wrists and fingers, legs, thighs, knees, calves, ankles and toes. It also stimulates fresh blood to the lower abdominal region. It is so wonderful for women because it helps to remove flab and cellulite from the top of the thighs. When you first try it, you may think your arms will never match up and as for your legs – impossible! – but keep practicing and you will realise its beauty. It is difficult at first, but you will be thrilled with the speed at which your stiffness disappears and also by the lovely shape of your legs!

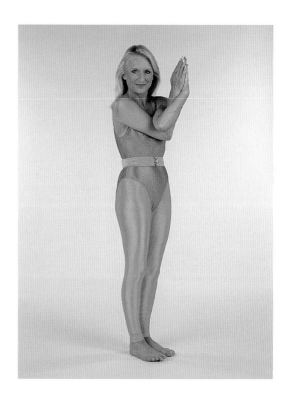

● Stand straight with your arms out in front of you. Cross the left upper arm over the right, and bring it under the right arm so that the hands are placed together in prayer position. Now interlock your fingers.

● Do the same with the legs. Cross the left thigh over the right, bending the right knee, then tuck the left foot around the right calf.

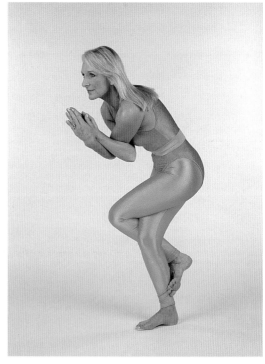

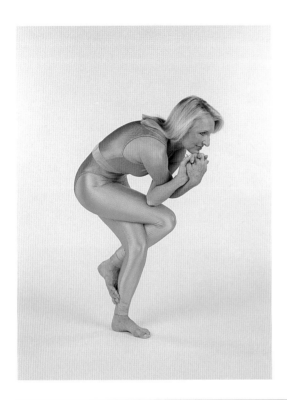

● Inhale then, as you exhale, bend forwards enabling you to place your lower elbow on your upper knee and resting your chin on your interlocked fingers. Hold for 5, breathing normally. Then inhale and return to a standing position and repeat to the other side. Repeat the entire sequence.

One of the benefits of this movement is to help remove cellulite. Along with other Yoga exercises, diet, deep breathing and relaxation techniques the stretching exercises really help tone the muscles for beautiful lean, firmer thighs. As we know, cellulite can be worsened by stress, so learning to relax is extremely beneficial. The Yoga diet helps to remove excess weight, and I recommend dry skin brushing every morning before you bathe to stimulate your circulation.

DRY SKIN BRUSHING

Buy a loofah or a natural body brush (my preference is for a loofah) and, every morning before you bathe, simply brush your body with even strokes in the direction of the heart. Do not brush over cuts or damaged skin and don't spend too long, about 2 minutes per day will do your whole body. This stimulates your circulation, exfoliates the skin and makes your skin glow. After bathing, pat yourself dry and moisturise your skin with your favourite fragrant moisturiser

CAT STRETCH

No self respecting cat would ever get up after a rest without stretching its spine carefully to make sure that it is fully flexible, tension free and ready for action. Our cat stretch does just that. It is excellent after rest, after a long car journey or after you have been shopping. It will help keep your spine beautifully mobile and is excellent for ridding it of stiffness and tension.

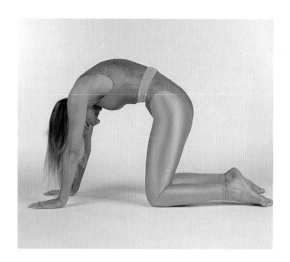

● Kneel down and place your hands on the floor in front of you so you are on all fours with your knees, feet and hands a foot apart. Slowly arch your back into a hump, dropping your head.

● Slowly lift your head and at the same time gently drop the lower back and stick your bottom out. Repeat this three times slowly and without strain. (Just doing this part of the exercise is great for removing tension from your spine and can really help an aching back.)

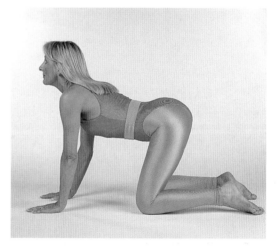

● Then gently bend the elbows and place your chin on the floor between your hands.

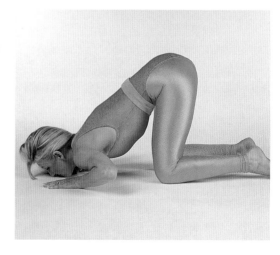

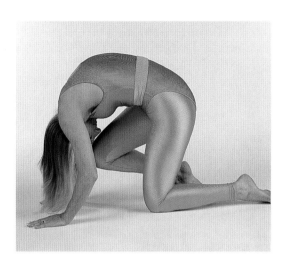

● Slowly straighten your arms and then take your right knee to your forehead.

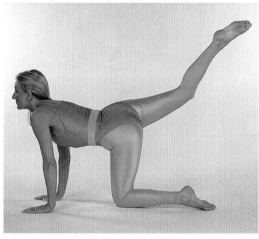

● Lift your head and look at the ceiling, then swing your right leg up and gently point your toes to the ceiling. Repeat this three times and then three times with the other leg. Gently lower your bottom to your heels, come up into a kneeling position and relax.

I am now entering my seventh month of pregnancy and have found that yoga has enabled me to remain relaxed, free of backache and unbelievably supple. I hope to continue with the classes until the baby is born and recommend it for any expectant mother.

A.H.

Having attended Barbara's classes for about a year, I only wish I had started Yoga earlier in my life. Inevitably one puts husbands/children/friends/jobs first and tears around everywhere with constant pressures and worries, forgetting that you need to look after your own mind and body in order to provide support for others.

I have found Yoga extremely beneficial in that it makes you more aware of your body and the importance of maintaining its flexibility. Yoga gives you a more positive attitude to life and helps you recognise stressful areas, not only in yourself but in family and friends and in so doing adopt a better, more balanced attitude to life.

S.H.

Since I have been doing Yoga my back has been fabulous! I am a nurse and do a lot of lifting in my job. Yoga has certainly strenghtened my muscles – no more backache!

S.N.

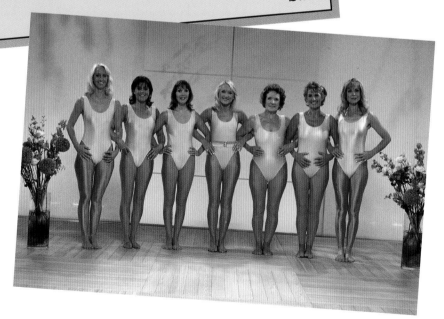

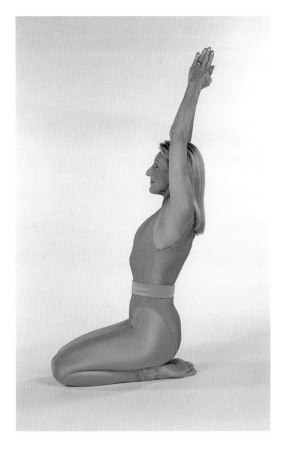

POSE OF A SWAN

This is a beautiful stretch for the spine and works really well after the Cat Stretch. It is a wonderful realigning stretch for the spine, increases the flexibility of the hips and is very relaxing.

● Kneel and place your bottom on your heels. Lift both arms in the air and inhale.

● As you exhale, stretch forwards and place your hands on the floor in front of you, but keep your bottom on your heels. Continue to stretch forwards into your maximum position and then relax in the movement and hold it, breathing normally, for a count of 10. Inhale and slowly return to an upright position and relax. There is no need to repeat this movement.

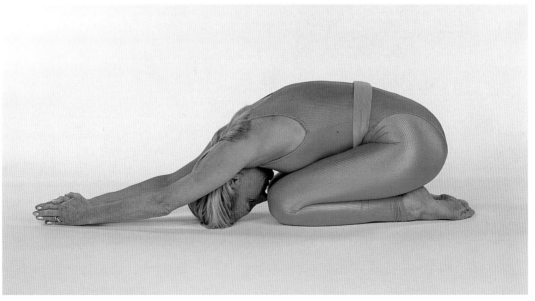

SIDEWAYS LEG RAISE

This movement firms the inner thighs, helps to remove cellulite, tones the buttocks and improves the flexibility of the hip joints.

● Lie on your left side, propped up on your left elbow.

● Breathe in, exhale and lift your right leg in the air.

● Clasp your right calf and try to draw your knee towards your ears. At first your hip will probably be a bit stiff but it will loosen as you practice so don't strain, just practice. Hold for a count of 5, then gently lower your leg. Repeat. Then repeat twice on the other side.

● Following this movement lie flat on the floor and draw your knees to your chest and, interlocking your hands around your knees, massage your back by rocking gently from side to side.

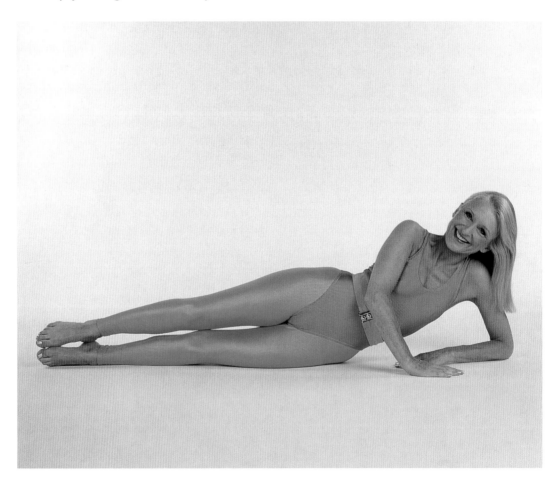

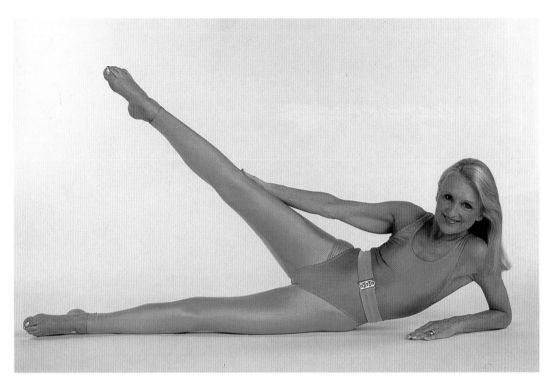

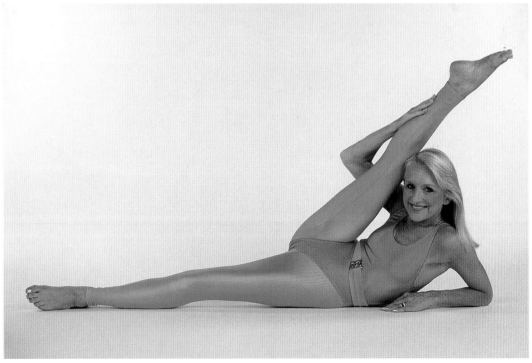

FULL TWIST

Once you have mastered the Simple Twist shown in Lesson Two (see p32), have a go at the Full Twist for that extra stretch. This really increases the circulation to the spinal nerves and increases the flexibility of the spine dramatically. It is also brilliant for slimming the waistline, hips and thighs, and toning the neck and abdominal organs.

● Sit straight with both legs straight out in front of you. Bring your left foot on to the floor between your legs, making sure the left knee is as near to the floor as possible.

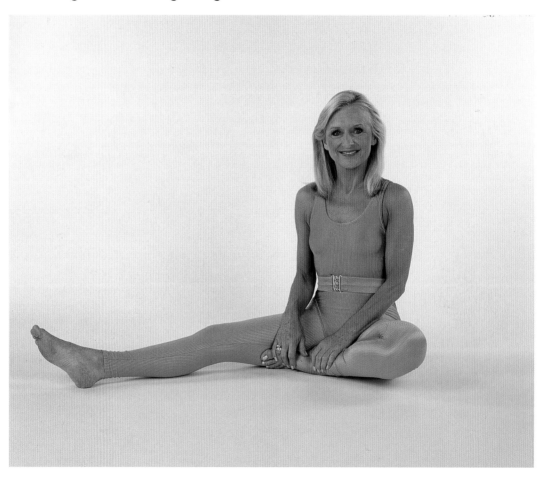

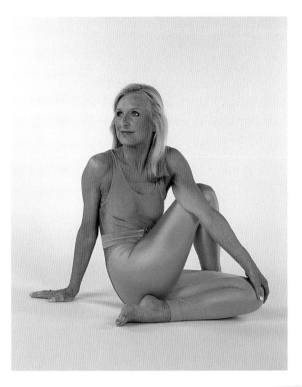

● Carefully lift your right leg and place it over your left thigh with your foot alongside your thigh and your knee high up. Place your right hand on the floor behind your back.

● Inhale then as you exhale place your left hand on the outside of your right knee and on your left knee and turn your head over your right shoulder and your whole torso to the right as much as possible without strain. Hold for a count of 5, then return your head to the front and repeat on the other side. Then repeat the entire routine.

I have started and given up many other forms of exercise but find that only Yoga gives me the sense of well-being and flexibility that I am looking for. I feel Yoga satisfies all the requirements of an exercise routine - it exercises all the muscles in the body without strain, including load-bearing exercises, so important for bones, as well as making me feel tension free and supple. I leave the classes with a 'spring in my step', feeling cheerful and positive, partly, I'm sure, due to Barbara's wonderful example of what Yoga can achieve and her sense of health and vitality.

H. H.

WIDE–ANGLED LEG STRETCH

This is a beautiful forwards stretch for the spine. It gently stretches the leg muscles and is wonderful for toning the inner thighs and calves. It might look difficult at first, but persevere and your body will feel fantastic. Remember *never* strain. This movement helps you to a really flexible back and thighs and keeps your legs in fabulous shape forever! It also great for your waistline. It stimulates the lower abdominal region and is a great help with menstrual problems.

● Sit straight with both legs very wide apart. (Don't worry they will widen as you continue to practice.) Place both arms parallel to your left leg.

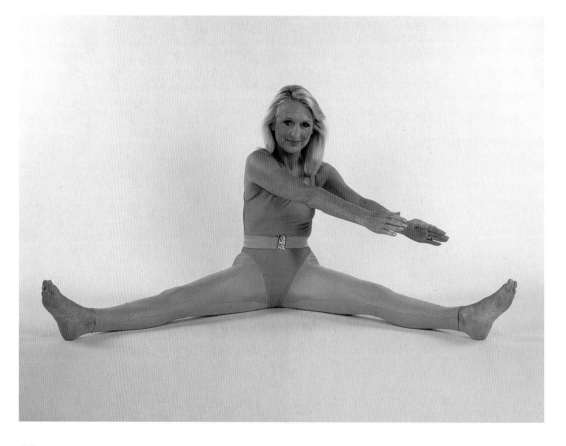

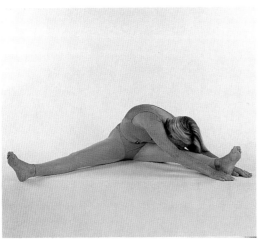

● Breathe in, then breathe out and slowly lean forwards, aiming to clasp the furthest part of your leg and taking your head towards your left knee. (Eventually you will clasp your ankle and take your head to your knee, but this will only come with practice.) Relax in this position for a count of 5, breathing normally, then lift the head, breathe in and slowly come up into a sitting position. Repeat to the other side.

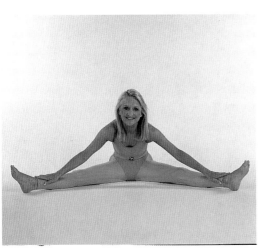

● Now place your hands on your upper thigh area. Breathe in and as you exhale, slowly slide your hands towards your ankles, keeping your back flat and your head up. Then slowly take your head towards the floor. Don't worry it won't come quickly, just do your best, half way is fine, don't strain, persevere.

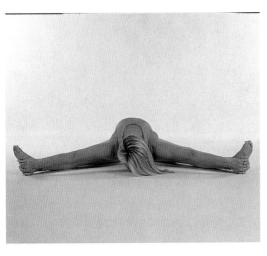

● Relax in your maximum position in this movement and then lift your head. Breathe in and slowly return to a sitting position and relax. Repeat.

WIDE–ANGLED PLOUGH

In Lesson Three we started to practice the Plough (see pp48-9). Here are some extra movements in this lovely exercise.

● Lie flat on your back. Inhale and gently lift your lower body off the floor, bending your knees and supporting your back with your hands as soon as the buttocks lift off. Exhale and allow your body to stretch into its maximum position without strain. When your feet can easily touch the floor behind you, open them as wide as possible for the Wide-Angled Plough and then take the hands back towards the feet. Relax in your maximum movement and hold for 30 seconds at first, gradually increasing the hold with practice. To come out of the pose slowly draw your legs together then bend the knees and very gently roll down your back, one vertebra at a time.

RELAXATION

Gently clasp your knees and rock your back from side to side. Then stretch both legs out in front of you and close your eyes and relax each muscle in turn.Now visualise a beautiful lake and see the surface of the lake is totally calm. Concentrate on the calm of the lake, just watch the surface, see the trees reflected in it, think calm and relax, relax, relax.

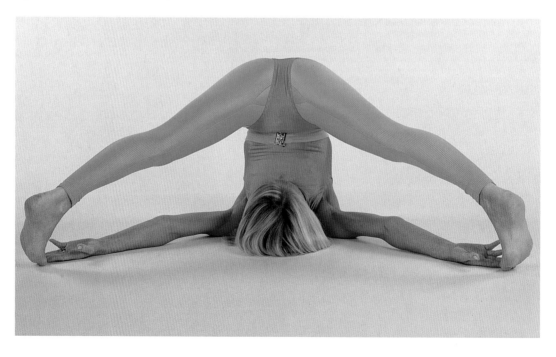

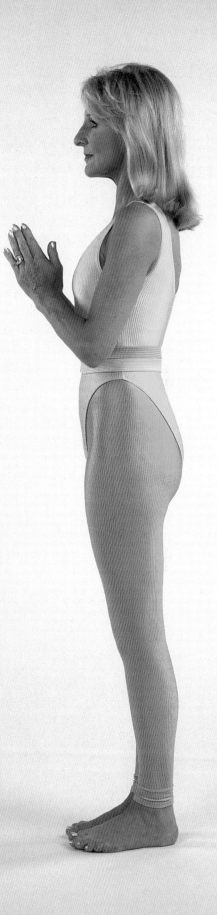

LESSON FIVE

Salute to the Sun
Triangle with Extra Movements
Wide-Angled Chest Expansion
Head to Knee Balance
Crescent Moon
Backwards Bend
Alternate Leg Pull
Thigh Stretch
Lotus Position
Relaxation

SALUTE TO THE SUN

This is a very beautiful exercise routine in 12 parts. Traditionally, it should be done facing the sunrise. The sun was worshiped in ancient times and thought to be the giver of health and immortal life. A totally energising routine, Salute to the Sun stretches, tones and firms the muscles in the arms and legs, reduces abdominal flab, and helps keep the spine flexible, promotes healthy deep breathing and helps the circulation. It really can do wonders for the whole body, maintaining that youthful flexibility and energy and keeping in it excellent shape.

Try to do the whole routine twice, alternating which leg you take back first in position 4. Once you have learned Salute to the Sun use it as an alternate morning stretch to the six super stretches you learned in Lesson One.

● Stand straight, feet together, breathe in deeply and exhale slowly.

● Raising your arms above your head, take a deep breath in and bend backwards. (Beginners may find it more comfortable to have the feet about 1 foot apart in this movement.)

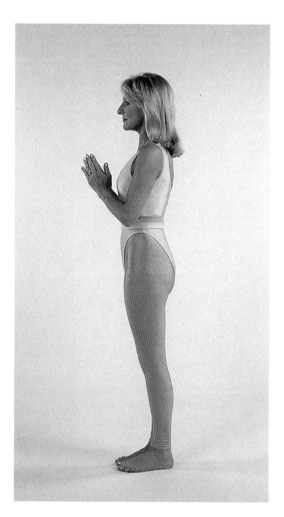

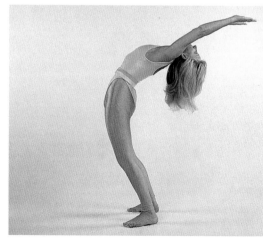

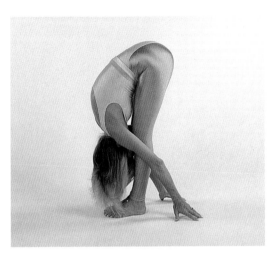

● Breathe out as you bend forwards, aiming your head to your knees and your hands by your feet. Aim to have the knees straight, but, if necessary, bend them in the beginning.

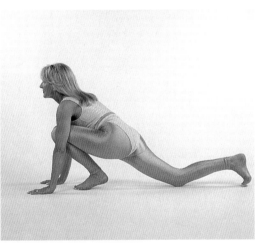

● Breathe in as you stretch your right leg back from your body, keeping the left leg between your hands, and look upwards.

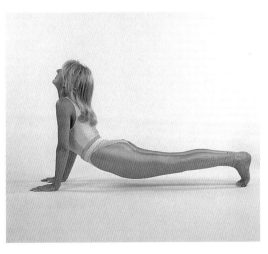

● Breathe out and stretch your left leg back.

● Lower the whole body to the floor. Knees first, then chest, then chin. Toes curled under.

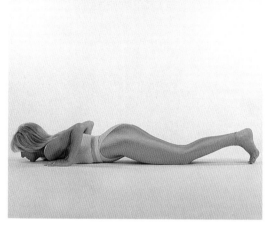

● Lie completely flat. Breathe in and slowly come up into the Cobra position, lifting your head, shoulders and upper body from the floor and dropping your head back.

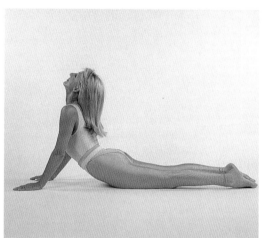

● Exhale and lift your bottom up in the air as you drop your head and shoulders, keeping your hands flat on the floor.

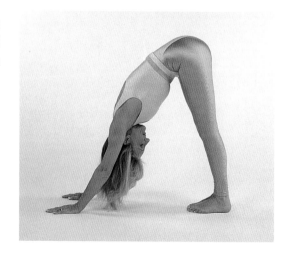

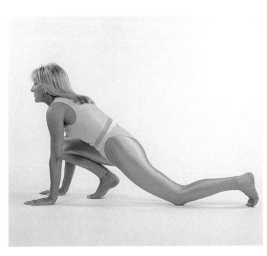

● Breathe in, and bring your right foot in between your hands and look up.

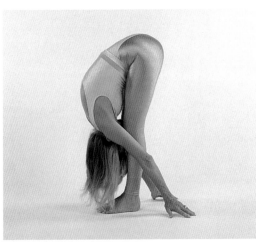

● Breathe out, bring your left foot in and look up. Then lift your bottom in the air and aim your head to your knees.

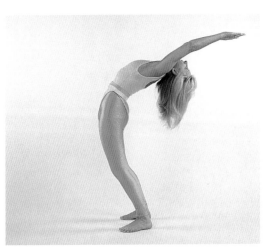

● Breathe in and slowly come up into an upright position raising your arms and bending backwards.

● Exhale, drop your arms and place them in prayer and relax.

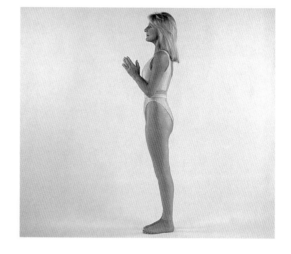

SALUTE TO THE SUN

Once you have learned this beautiful sequence, you will want to practice it daily, so here is the whole routine for your convenience

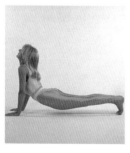 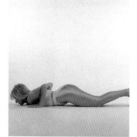 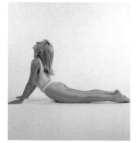 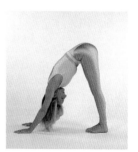

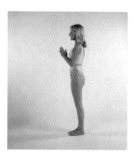 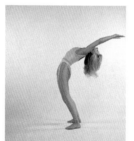 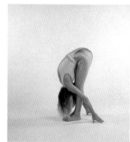 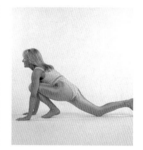

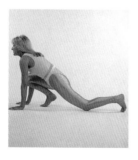 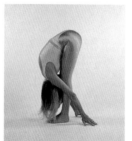 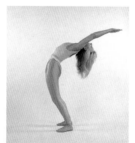 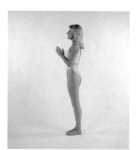

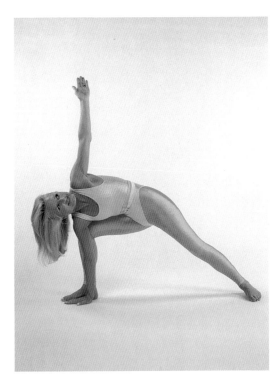

TRIANGLE WITH EXTRA MOVEMENTS

We first learned the Triangle in Lesson One (see p17). These extra stretches will gently increase your flexibility.

● Stand straight and place your legs about 4 feet apart. Turn your right foot to a 90 degree angle and lift your arms parallel to the floor. Take a deep breath and bend your right knee, aiming for your thigh to be flat, and gently lower your right hand towards your right foot, as in Lesson One. Exhale and lift your left arm in the air pulling your shoulder back and pointing your fingers to the ceiling. Turn your head to look at the ceiling. Hold the position for a count of 5, breathing normally. Then inhale and return to an upright position and repeat on the other side.

● Now, for that extra stretch, with your arms parallel to the floor, swap your arms over, placing the left thumb by your right big toe and pointing your right arm to the ceiling. Hold the position for a count of 5 breathing normally. Inhale and return to an upright position and repeat to the other side.

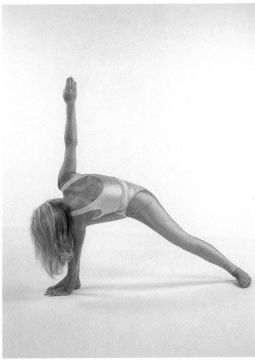

WIDE–ANGLED CHEST EXPANSION

This movement firms the buttocks, calves and thighs and is excellent for the upper arms and bust. It is a great stress reliever, loosens the shoulders and corrects poor posture and is also good for relieving tightness in the chest.

● Standing with your feet about 3-4 feet apart, inhale and stretch your arms up high, then slowly bend forwards with your back flat and your head up and move into your maximum position without strain. Now take your arms back behind you and interlock your fingers. Pull your arms up as high as possible, keeping the elbows straight, and relax in your maximum position breathing normally. Hold for a count of 5 then, lifting your head slowly, inhale and return to an upright position. Eventually your head may reach the floor, but please don't strain, gently does it!

● With a full lung, pull your arms back under your bottom and bend backwards, relaxing back as you exhale. Inhale and return to an upright position, then gently exhale, lower your arms and relax. Repeat once.

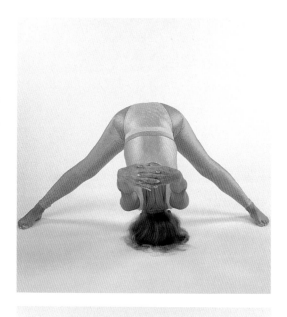

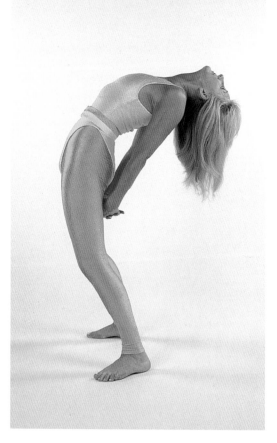

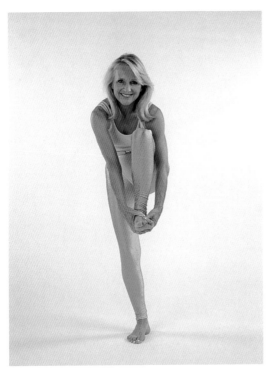

HEAD TO KNEE BALANCE

Once you have mastered this movement and held it for a count of 5, you know that you can do almost anything! It gives you amazing confidence and flexibility. It is wonderful for the backs of the thighs and calves. It strengthens the legs and is excellent for concentration. It appears very difficult at first, but once you have mastered it you seem to have it forever.

● Standing straight, inhale and bend your left knee, clasping your left foot in both hands.

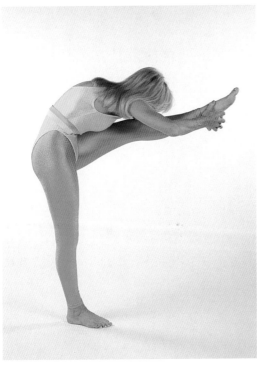

● Now, with your right leg straight, inhale, straighten your left leg and gently lower your chin to your knee. Focus on a spot to help your concentration and hold for a count of 5, breathing normally. It is not easy at first to straighten the leg, but it will come with practice. Inhale, lower your leg to the floor, straighten up and relax. Repeat on the other side.

CRESCENT MOON

This beautiful movement is excellent for relieving tensions in the shoulders. It firms the thighs, hips, abdomen and throat and once you have mastered it you receive a beautiful, warm flow of peace and relaxed energy.

● Adopt a high kneeling position. Place your left foot in front of you and extend your right leg back, stretching it as straight as possible. Push your left buttock towards your left foot. Inhale and lift both arms in the air.

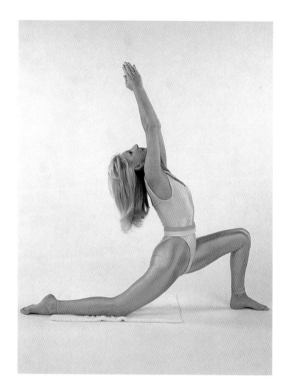

● Slowly and gently stretch back. It might not be far at first, but your stretch will increase as you practice. Hold for 5, breathing normally, then inhale and return to an upright position and relax. Repeat on the other side. Then repeat on both sides.

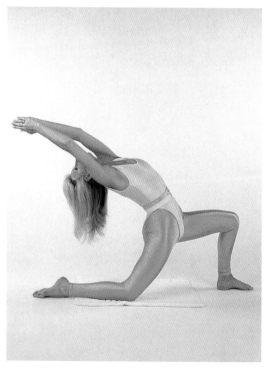

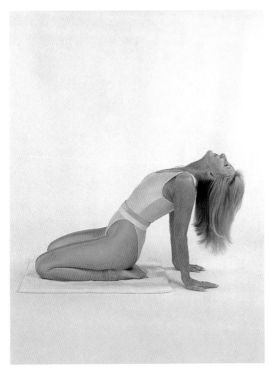

BACKWARDS BEND

A great de-stresser, the Backwards Bend tones the thighs, helps keep the chest and throat in perfect condition and it is a beautiful backwards stretch for the spine and chest area.

● Sit on your heels and place your hands on the floor underneath your shoulders, fingers pointing backwards.

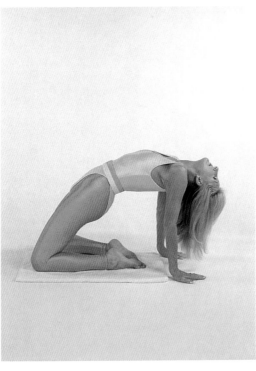

● Inhale and lift your bottom as high as possible from your heels. (Don't worry if it is difficult. Don't strain. Keep practicing and, gradually, you will improve.) Exhale and hold for a count of 5, breathing normally, then gently lower your bottom to your heels and inhaling lean forwards. Exhale, place your head in front of your knees and your arms by your sides and relax in the Pose of a Child. Hold this for a few seconds, and then slowly return to a kneeling position. Repeat once.

ALTERNATE LEG PULL

We first tried this in Lesson Three (see p47).

● Sit straight with both legs straight out in front of you. Lift your right foot on to your left thigh and gently bounce the flexed knee up and down to loosen your knee, hip and ankle. If your foot feels comfortable on your upper thigh and your right knee is close to the ground, leave it on your thigh for a slightly stronger stretch. If not, rest your foot next to your thigh. Don't strain. Inhale and lift both arms parallel to the outstretched leg. Then lift both arms straight up in the air.

● Exhale and stretch forwards clasping the leg gently or putting your hands on the floor by the sides of your foot and eventually aiming your chin to your knee. Hold and relax in your maximum position, starting at a count of 5 and gradually increasing to 10 as your flexibility improves. Inhale and slowly return to an upright position. Relax and repeat. Repeat twice on the other side.

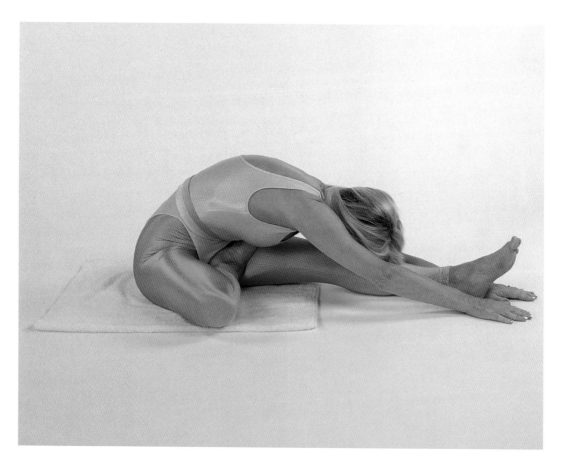

THIGH STRETCH

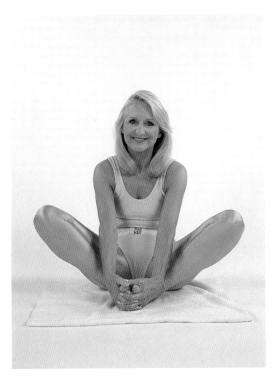

This movement tones the inner thigh area and keeps the hip joint really supple. Your body will respond quickly to this movement. Never be discouraged if you are initially stiff – once your hips have regained that youthful flexibility your walk will look 10 years younger!

● Sit very straight and bring both feet towards your body, placing the soles of your feet together and clasping them in both hands.

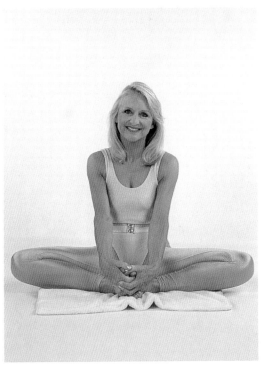

● Breathe in, then breathe out and gently lower your knees to the floor. Hold your maximum position in this movement for a count of 5, breathing normally, then slowly return your knees to their upright position and relax. Repeat this movement 3 times.

LOTUS POSITION

Once your hips, ankles and knees are sufficiently flexible, try the Lotus Position. With practice, this movement improves the flexibility and health of your knees, ankles, hips and feet. Always remember: never force this position. Most movements can be done in an easy cross-legged position and your progress in Yoga does *not* depend on your ability to do the Lotus position.

● Sit with your legs crossed. Carefully lift your right foot on to your left thigh for the Half Lotus position.

● When the Half Lotus is easy and comfortable, then carefully try to lift your left foot on to your right thigh for the Full Lotus. This may take some time – and after that it does take a while for it to become comfortable. But it is the perfect sitting position. Your back is straight and it is ideal for breathing exercises. You feel calm and focused. As you progress, your legs will feel better and better. Alternate the legs in this position every time you try it.

RELAXATION

Do remember to lie down and relax – this time, try to visualise a beautiful, clear night sky. Relax each muscle in turn, slow your breathing down and see the full moon shining on the ocean. Stay relaxed for 5-10 minutes, then take a deep breath, refreshed and ready to tackle anything!

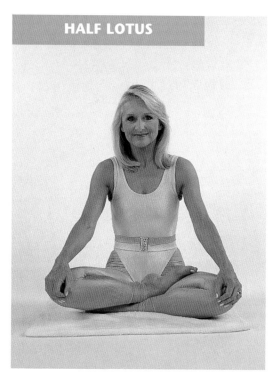

HALF LOTUS

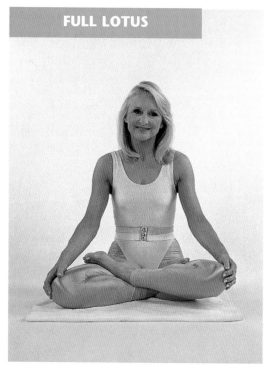

FULL LOTUS

80

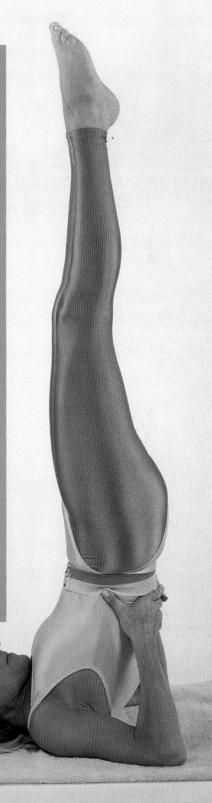

LESSON SIX

Sleeping Time Sequence

This is one of my favourite sequences to alleviate stress and aid relaxation and sleep. To make it a perfect morning routine simply precede it with Salute to the Sun (see pages 68-72).

**Cat Stretch
Bar of a Gate
Camel
Pose of a Cow
Pose of a Frog
Alternate Nostril Breathing
Exercise
Sit Up Lie Down
Chest Expansion – Kneeling
Head and Neck Exercises
Shoulderstand
Pose of a Fish
Relaxation**

CAT STRETCH

We first learned this movement in Lesson Four (see pp56-7).

● Kneel and place your hands on the floor in front of you so you are on all fours. Place your knees, feet and hands a foot apart and slowly arch your back into a hump, dropping your head. Slowly lift your head and at the same time gently drop your lower back and stick your bottom out. Repeat this three times slowly and without strain.

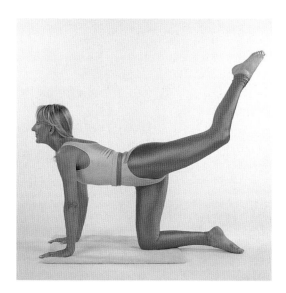

● Gently bend your elbows and place your chin on the floor between your hands. Slowly straighten your arms and then take your left knee to your forehead. Lift your head and look at the ceiling and at the same time lift your left leg and point your toe to the ceiling. Repeat this three times and then three times with the other leg.

● After this movement, realign your spine with the Pose of a Swan (see p59).

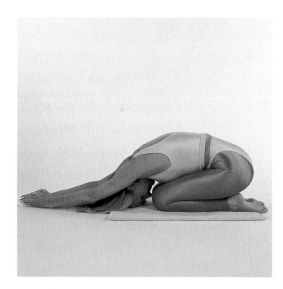

82

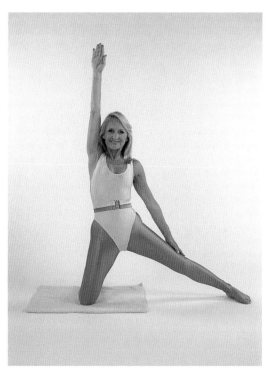

BAR OF A GATE

This lovely movement is excellent for toning the waistline, abdomen and inner thighs. It is also very good for relieving stiffness and tension in the lower back.

● Kneel in an upright position and place your left foot out to the side, keeping your right knee on the floor. Inhale and lift your right arm.

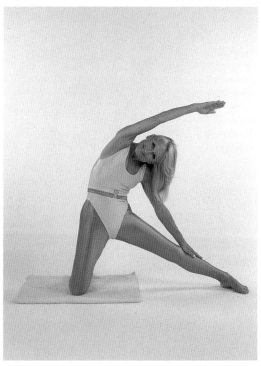

● Exhaling, gradually slide your left hand down your left leg stretching your right arm over your head as far as possible. Hold for a count of 5, breathing normally, then inhale and return to an upright position. Lower the arm and relax. Repeat on the other side and then repeat the whole sequence twice.

THE CAMEL

We first learned this movement in Lesson Two (see pp30-31). It's marvellous for relieving tension, your cares just float away!

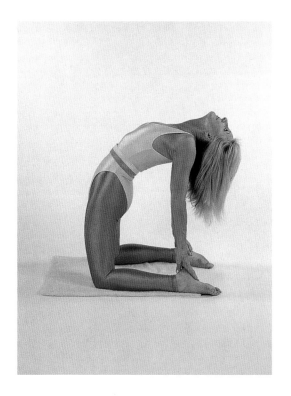

● Adopt a high kneeling position with your hands at your waistline, thumbs in front and fingers behind, knees and feet 1 foot apart. Breathe in deeply and allow your upper body to bend backwards, keeping your thighs straight. Exhale once you have reached your maximum position.

If you can, place your right hand on your right foot and your left hand on your left foot. If you can't just keep your hands at your waistline and hold your maximum position for a count of 5 breathing normally. Inhale as your return to an upright position.

Exhale and allow your bottom to sink to your heels with your hands by your sides and your head on the floor in the Pose of a Child and relax for a count of 5. Breathe in, and return to a kneeling position and repeat the sequence twice.

For me, Yoga proved that exercise didn't have be painful! I like it because you really feel that you can do it at your own pace, in a non-competitive environment.

R.G.

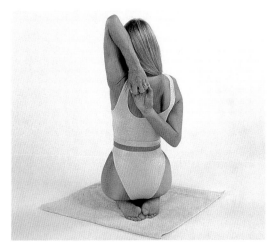

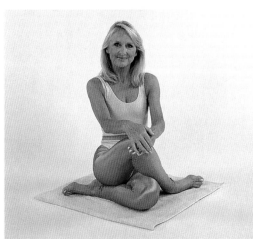

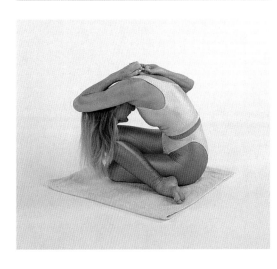

POSE OF A COW

I seriously urge you to start practicing this movement. Nowadays, with the pressures and hectic speed of modern life, it is easy to acquire stiffness in the shoulder area. This brilliant movement helps prevent restrictions and pain in the shoulders. It also helps to lift the bust, tones the underarm area and prevents poor posture.

● Adopt a comfortable kneeling position and, lifting your left arm in the air, drop it behind your back. Take your right arm behind your back and try to link your hands. Hold, undo and relax, then repeat on the other side. Don't worry, this can be very difficult, to begin with you may use a belt or a tie to help you. When you are comfortable in the arm movement try this pose in the correct, slightly more difficult, position which is wonderful for your thighs.

● Adopt a high kneeling position. Cross your right leg over your left, spread your feet out and very carefully place your bottom between your heels. Do not strain, if you a find this difficult simply return to a kneeing position.

● Then lift your left arm and drop it behind your back and take your right hand behind your back to join. Inhale deeply then exhale and carefully draw your head to your upper knee. Hold for 5, relax and return to an upright position. Repeat on the other side.

85

POSE OF A FROG

This is excellent for removing tension from your lower back, toning your inner thighs and maintaining joint mobility in the hip area.

● From a kneeling position open the thighs and stretch the knees apart really wide. Place one set of toes over the other, or let the toes just touch. Place your bottom on your heels.

● Take a large breath and as you exhale stretch forward, opening your arms wide apart. Aim to place your chin on the floor, keeping your bottom on your heels.

● Relax in the position, holding for a count of 10, breathing normally. Then inhale and return slowly to an upright position, exhale and relax. There is no need to repeat.

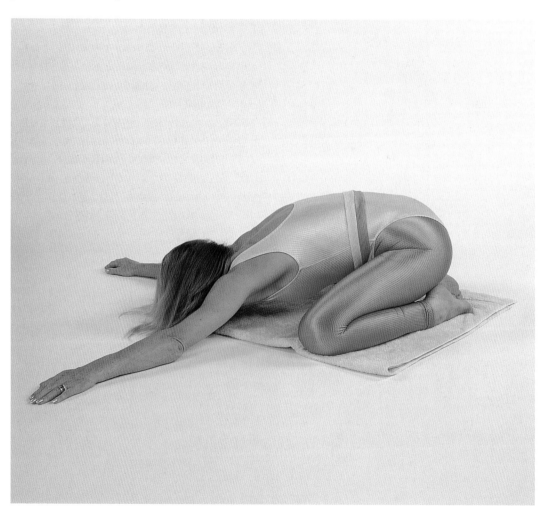

ALTERNATE NOSTRIL BREATHING EXERCISE

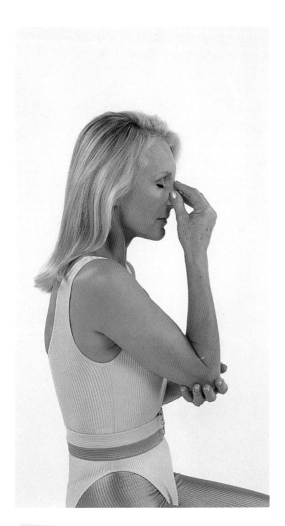

This is perfect after an upsetting situation, when you feel hassled, when you are under stress and anytime you wish to calm yourself down. It is a relaxing breath and makes you feel serene, calm and able to cope. Remember, tension is ageing! This is a brilliant tranquilliser anytime, but is especially beneficial before sleep.

● Sit in a comfortable position with your back straight. Place your right thumb on your right nostril, the next 2 fingers on the bridge of your nose and the next finger on your left nostril. Unblock the right nostril by lifting the thumb and inhale for a count of 5. Hold the breath for 5 then block the right nostril, unblock the left and exhale through the left nostril for 5. Inhale left and hold. Exhale right. Inhale right and hold. Exhale left. Do 10 rounds altogether.

I have been doing Yoga for over two years now and it has completely transformed my life. When I started I was tense, suffered regular panic attacks and had a huge guilt complex about doing anything 'for me'. I learned to relax, got a much better figure and now have a little more time for myself. I often use the things we have learned when I find everyday life taking over and they really do help. I cannot recommend Yoga highly enough - it really does make sense.

S.P.

SIT UP LIE DOWN

This is brilliant after a hard day. It tones the spine, firms the tum and thighs and is a totally beautiful relaxing stretch. It is done in a continuous motion, no holds, and is a perfect 'before bed' relaxing routine, for those times when one just can't switch off. After this you sleep like a baby!

● Lie flat on the floor, arms flat and straight behind your head. Inhale and return to a sitting position. (If this is difficult, use your arms to help you up at first.) Exhale as you move into back-stretch just as far as you can without strain. Inhale as you return to a sitting position.

● Exhale as you lie flat on the floor. Slowly does it! Inhale and lift your legs (bending your knees if necessary).

● Exhale as you stretch back into the Plough position. Just go as far as you can with no strain. Slowly roll down and flow into backstretch. Never strain in any of the movements. Repeat 5 times. Then gently draw your knees to your chest and rock your back from side to side.

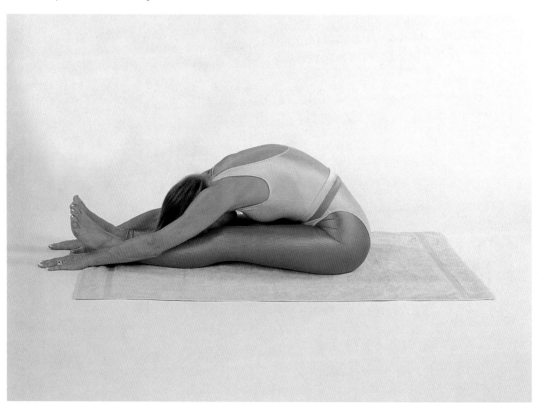

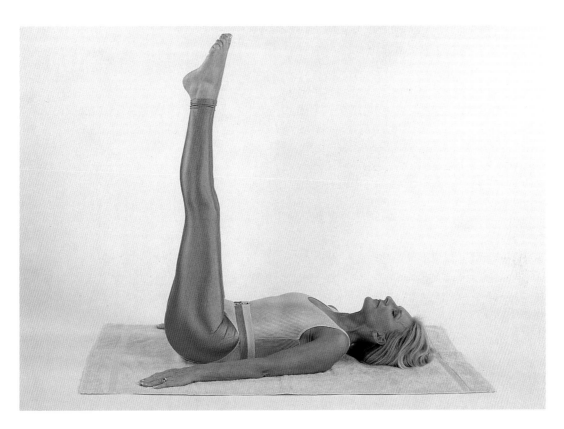

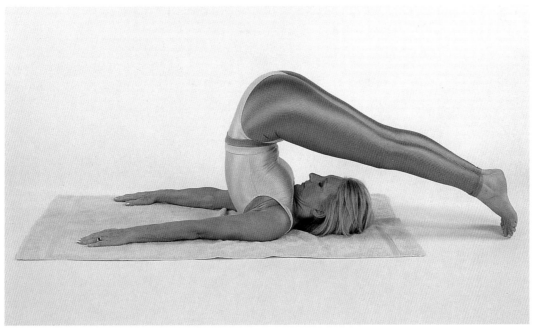

CHEST EXPANSION – KNEELING

We first tried the Chest Expansion in Lesson Two (see pp24-5). This movement, in a kneeling position, relaxes the muscles at the back of the shoulders, as well as toning your upper arms and firming your bust. The results are amazing and you will feel and look relaxed and comfortable.

● Kneel and interlock your hands behind your back, keeping your elbows straight. Inhale and raise your arms as high as possible, holding for a count of 5.

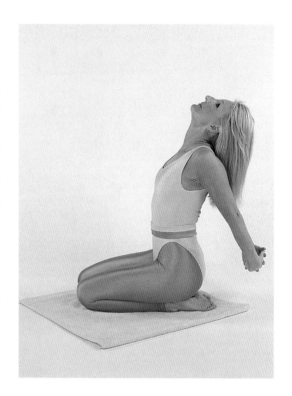

● Exhale and gently lower your head to the floor and continuing to lift your arms. Hold the position for a count of 5, breathing normally. Inhale and return to an upright kneeling position. Hold for 5 with your arms still high, then relax your arms and you should experience a lovely warm glow as the shoulder and neck muscles relax. Repeat 3 times.

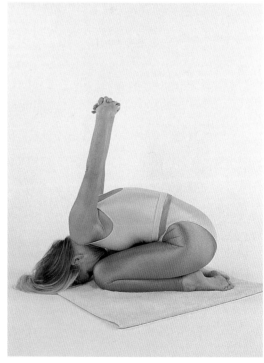

90

HEAD AND NECK EXERCISES

CAUTION: If you have problems with your neck do consult your doctor before doing the head and neck exercises.

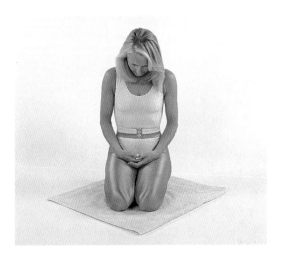

This exercise tones the muscles in the neck and throat and relaxes the muscles at the base of the neck which are susceptible to stiffness. This is beneficial if performed last thing at night, and is recommended for headache and migraine sufferers. When I started teaching Yoga 25 years ago, this movement was enjoyed by all. Nowadays necks are a different matter. They are often stiff and tense, so I urge you to be careful. At first your neck may only be able to move to move half an inch each way. To start with, expand the circle as your neck begins to improve – always go very gently, *never strain*. These movements help correct double chin and restore flexibility. Nothing ruins your skin and the way you look and feel more than tension, so do try to use these exercises when under stress.

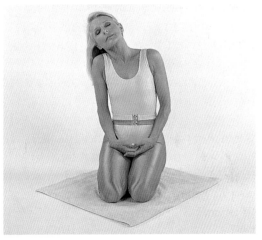

● Sit in a comfortable cross-legged or kneeling position, making sure your spine is straight. Gently drop your head forwards, then slowly roll it to the right, then slowly backwards, slowly to the left and then slowly forwards so your head is making a gentle circling movement. Try to do 4 circles to the right, then 4 to the left.

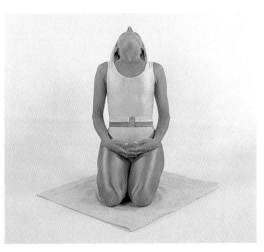

SHOULDERSTAND

CAUTION: This exercise must not be done if you suffer from high blood pressure or any problem in the head and neck area.

For ages Yoga has been renowned by film stars as the best method for keeping the body young and flexible and reducing the ageing effects caused by lack of muscle tone and a general drooping and sagging of the body. The shoulderstand increases the circulation to the head and neck area, benefiting the skin, hair and brain cells. It is excellent for people who suffer from varicose veins and haemorrhoids. It stimulates the thyroid and parathyroid glands in the neck, and will help to rejuvenate the spine and strengthen and firm the muscles of the back, legs, neck and abdomen.

● Lie flat on your back with your hands relaxed by your sides, palms down. Breathe in deeply, then breathe out and, bending your knees, slowly lift your legs and buttocks off the floor. Keep lifting them until you reach your own maximum position, supporting your back by placing your hands at your waistline. Eventually your body will be completely straight, but do be patient as this will only come with practice and you will still benefit in the early stages of the exercise. To begin with, hold the

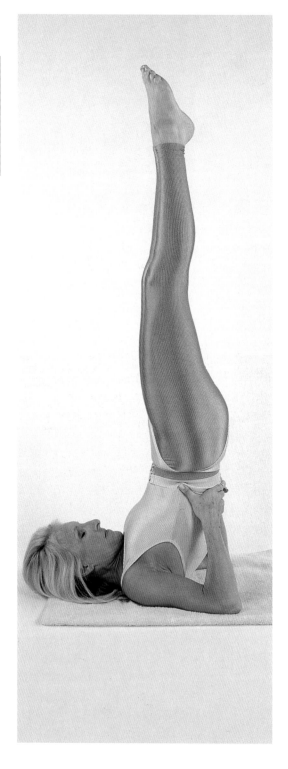

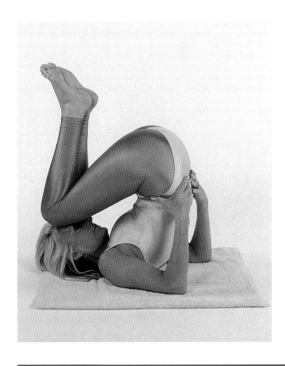

position for a maximum of 30 seconds. Gradually, over a period of six months, increase the hold as you practice it until you are holding for about 3 minutes.

● To come out of the Shoulderstand, draw your knees to your forehead, then very slowly roll down your back one vertebra at a time until your bottom touches the floor. Interlock your hands around your knees and rock your back from left to right. Then slowly let your legs go straight out in front of you and relax.

Yoga and the Beautiful Body

By now I am sure you are seeing the results of your Yoga practice. Yoga will realign you, balance the imbalanced parts of your body and relieve tension throughout.

In my opinion, of any exercise system, Yoga gives you the most beautiful body shape for your particular size and frame. It creates long, lean, beautiful muscles, it whittles the waistline, it firms the thighs and upper arms and gently coaxes all parts of your body into the best shape for you.

There is simply nothing we leave out in Yoga. The inverted postures are excellent for the skin and hair and renewal of energy; joints are made flexible; all muscles are toned and made lean; abdominals and chins are firmed. In all, the body acquires beautiful shape and balance at any age.

POSE OF A FISH

This beautiful movement is excellent for relaxing the neck and chest. It is very beneficial for asthma sufferers and a great boon before sleep, as it is an excellent tension reliever for the upper body.

● Lie flat on your back and place your hands under your buttocks, palms down, with your elbows on the floor. Inhale and lift the head and shoulders, arching your upper body. Now gently bring the top of your head to the floor. Breathe normally in the position, hold for a count of 10, then lower your body to the floor, place your arms palms up and relax.

RELAXATION

At this stage, depending on the time of day, if you wish, just get straight into bed or lie on the floor, making sure you are warm enough. Have your feet about 2-3 feet apart, your arms palms up and about 1 foot from the body. Then go through your body systematically relaxing each muscle in turn until your whole body feels warm and really relaxed. Feel comfortable, slow your breathing down and now visualise a beautiful clear night sky and fill it with a thousand stars. Just see the vastness of the universe. Keep it in your mind and relax, relax, relax.

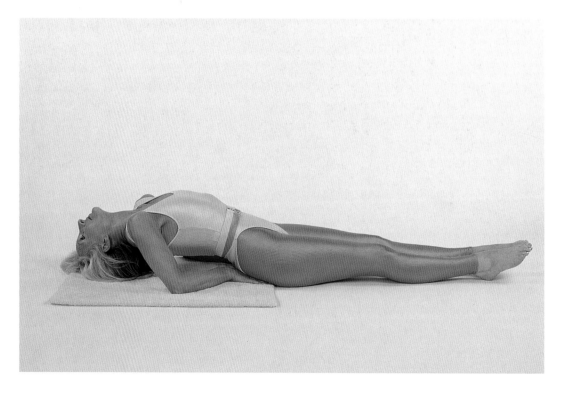

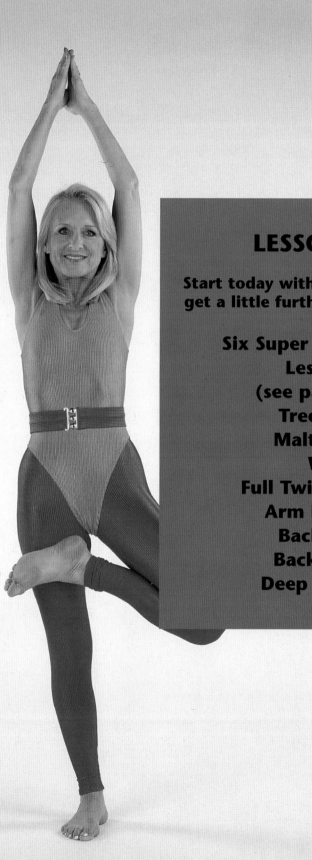

LESSON SEVEN

Start today with Lesson One, trying to get a little further in each movement.

**Six Super Stretches from
Lesson One
(see pages 12-20)
Tree Balance
Maltese Cross
Wheel
Full Twist with Extra
Arm Movement
Back Stretch
Back Roll and
Deep Relaxation**

TREE BALANCE

We first learned this movement in Lesson Two (see p28). Here are some extra stretches for you to try. This lovely balance breaks down into 3 stages, but always go gently, do a tiny bit each day – *don't* strain.

Stage One

● Stand straight and place your left foot on your right thigh. Breathe in and lift your arms above your head and stretch. Hold for a count of 5, increasing to a count of 10 as your confidence grows. Lower your arms and leg, relax and repeat on the other side.

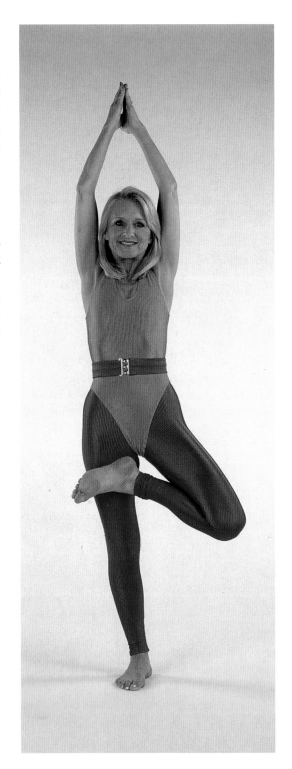

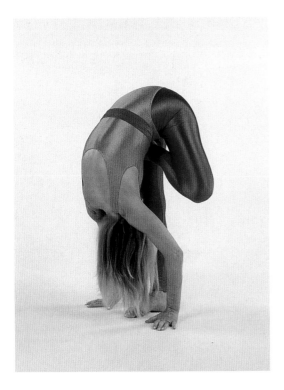

Stage Two

● Place your left foot on your right thigh. Inhale and stretch upwards, then exhale and lower your arms down to touch the floor and gently draw your head to your knee. Then inhale and slowly lift your head concentrate on a spot to help you balance, and slowly return to an upright position. Relax and repeat on the other side.

Note: this is a strong stretch. You might not get very far down at first. That's OK. Just start with a few inches forwards and then come up again, gradually increasing the movement each time you practice it. Only when you can do Stage Two with ease may you move on to Stage Three.

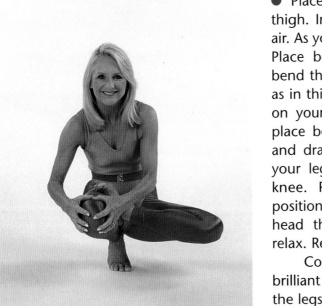

Stage Three

● Place your left foot on your right thigh. Inhale and lift both arms in the air. As you exhale gently bend forwards. Place both hands on the floor, then bend the right leg and aim to balance, as in this photograph, with both hands on your front knee. Hold for 5. Now place both hands on the floor. Inhale and draw your bottom up, straighten your leg and aim your head to your knee. Return slowly to a standing position. Stretch your arms above your head then place them together and relax. Repeat on the other side.

Congratulations! This movement is brilliant for all the muscles and joints of the legs – well worth the effort.

MALTESE CROSS

This series is excellent for firming your abdominals, trimming the waistline and firming the thighs. These 3 movements are among my favourites. They will help keep your hips flexible and free from stiffness.

Stage One

This movement will gradually increase the flexibility while toning the inner thigh muscles.

● Lie flat on your back with your arms outstretched, palms up.

● Carefully move your right foot towards your right hand. Keep the foot on the floor. Hold in your maximum position, then carefully return the foot to the starting position again and relax. Repeat on the other side. Don't worry about how little your leg moves in the beginning, move without strain and, as you practice, one day the foot will touch the hand. Repeat twice on each side.

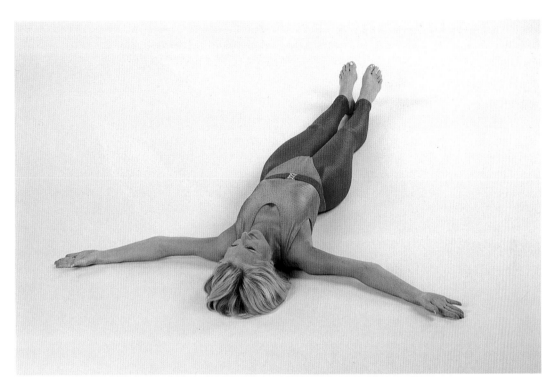

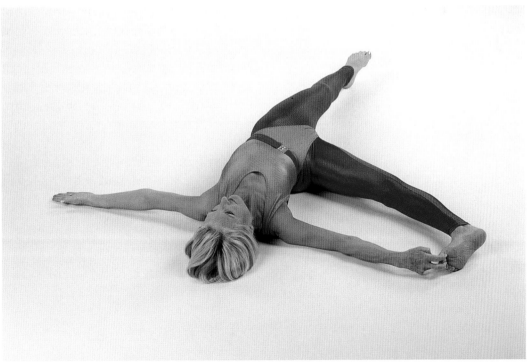

MALTESE CROSS

Stage Two

This is excellent for firming your abdominals and thighs and trimming the waistline.

● Lie flat on your back with your arms outstretched, palms up.

I started Yoga at the age of 50, with a somewhat old and rusty body! Now, after going reguarly for three years, I am looking forward to retiring at 95, with no tupperware hips, no dowager's hump and being able to hop in and out of a little red Ferrari.

W.A.

● Inhale and lift your left leg and, exhaling, gently take it towards your right hand. (Again, do your best, the hip will quickly acquire more flexibility.) Hold in your maximum position for a count of 5, then inhale lift the left leg keeping it straight and exhale slowly and lower it to the floor. Repeat on the other side. Repeat twice.

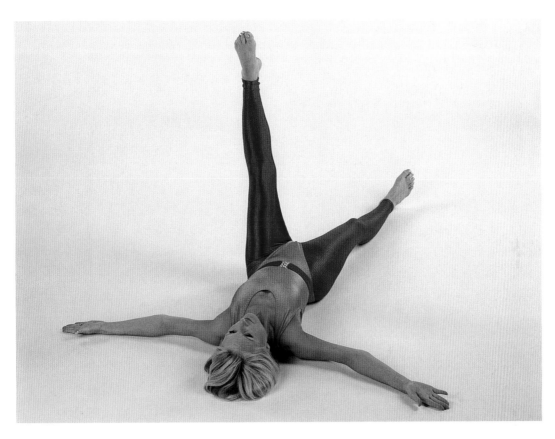

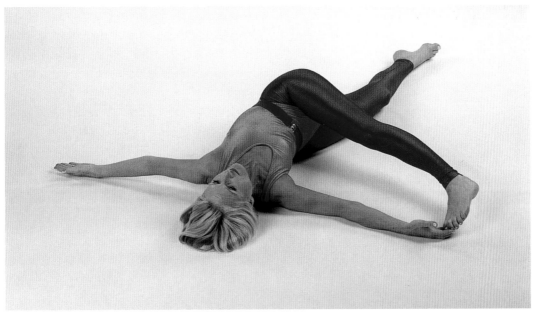

MALTESE CROSS

Stage Three

This movement is excellent for the backs of the legs. It also tones the front of the thighs and is a superb abdominal firmer.

● Lie flat on your back.

● Inhale and lift your left leg in the air. Using both hands grasp your leg and, carefully lifting the upper body a little, exhale and draw your left knee to your nose or as far as is possible without strain. Hold, then lower the leg and head carefully to the floor. Repeat on the other side and repeat the entire sequence twice.

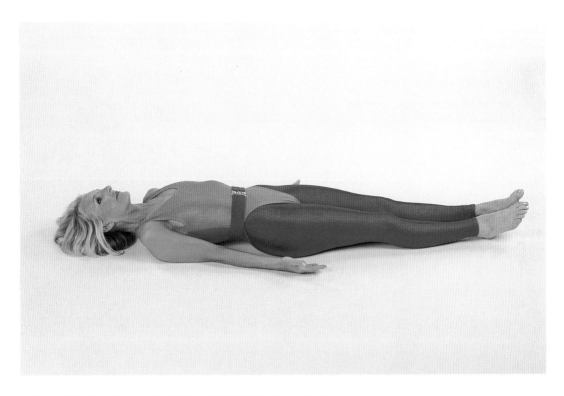

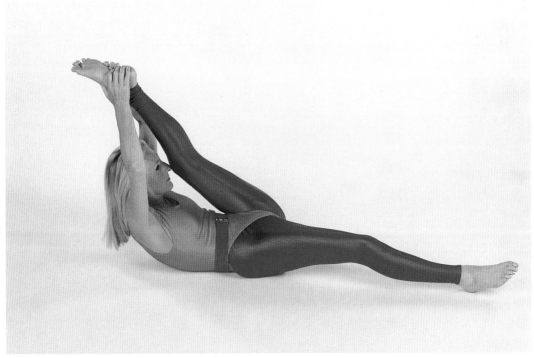

THE WHEEL

Yoga's ultimate backwards stretch. Most of us did this as children – but why did we stop? It is great for energising the entire body and keeping your spine flexible for life. I have put all the stages in this exercise but please progress at your own pace. This is wonderful for firming the bottom and abdomen and strengthening the lower back. You *can* do this and it will help you to regain amazing flexibility. I have many pupils who do this for the first time in their lives in their 60s and 70s – It's never too late!

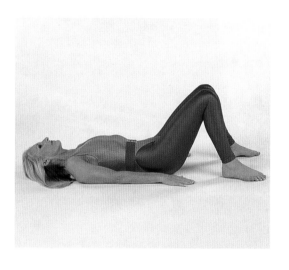

Stage One

● Lie flat on your back, arms by your sides. Inhale and as you exhale lift only your buttocks from the floor. Tighten them, hold for a count of 5 then relax. Repeat 3 times.

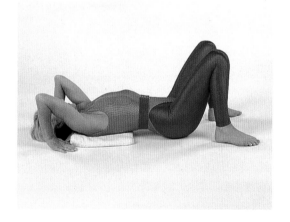

Stage Two

Lie flat on the floor placing your hands by your shoulders, fingers pointing into the shoulders. Place your feet flat on the floor, about 1 foot apart. Inhale and as you exhale lift your body and rest your head on the floor. Hold and then slowly lower your body to the floor. Draw your knees to your chest and gently rock your back from side to side to relax it. When your confidence increases, try to fold your arms on your chest for a stronger stretch.

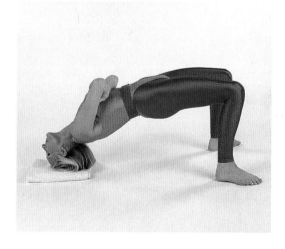

Stage Three

When you have managed Stage Two comfortably then *and only then* may you try the Wheel.

Lie on the floor, hands by your shoulders, fingers pointing into your shoulders, palms flat, feet about 1 foot apart and knees bent. Inhale deeply and as you exhale lift the entire body from the floor. (A little tip: try to think only of lifting your head and straightening your arms.)

Eventually try to straighten your arms and legs and push up as high as possible. Then, breathing normally in the position, try to hold for a count of 5, lengthening the hold as you progress in the movement. Then slowly lower your body down to the floor, draw your knees to your chest and gently rock your back from side to side and relax.

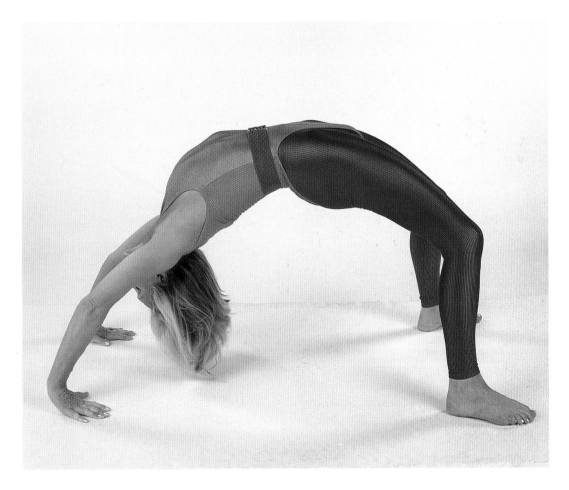

FULL TWIST WITH EXTRA ARM MOVEMENT

Once you have mastered the Simple Twist in Lesson Two (see p32) and had a go at the Full Twist for that extra stretch in Lesson Four (see pp62-3), now try the Full Twist with a small extra movement to help the flexibility of the shoulders.

● Sit straight with both legs straight out in front of you. Bend your left knee, bringing the foot on to the floor in the middle between your legs. Make sure your left knee is as near to the floor as possible.

● Carefully lift your right leg and place it over your left leg, with your foot alongside your thigh and the knee high up.

● Place your right hand on the floor behind your back. Inhale then, as you exhale, take your left arm outside your right knee and place your hand on your left knee, turning your head over your right shoulder.

● Now take your left hand carefully under your right knee and take your right hand behind your back and try to join them. It will take time. Don't strain. Hold for a count of 5, then undo your hands return your head to the front and repeat on the other side. Then repeat the entire routine.

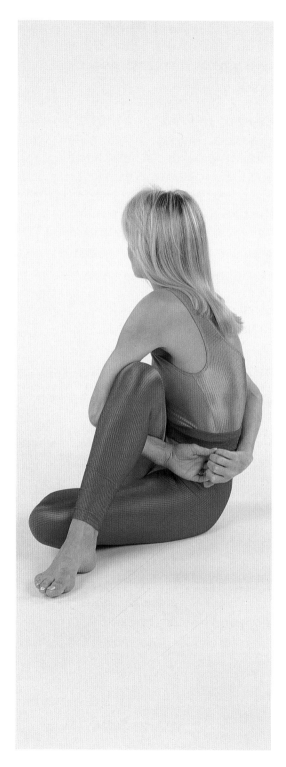

BACK STRETCH

We first practiced this movement in Lesson Two (see p33). Now try and stretch a little more. Every time you practice this movement you will gain in flexibility. Remember, the Back Stretch is excellent for toning the backs of the thighs and helping to remove abdominal flab as well as realigning the spine.

● Sit straight with both legs straight out in front of you. Breathe in and slowly stretch your arms up as high as possible. Exhale and stretch forwards without strain.

● Clasp your legs or place your hands on the floor and gently lower your chin to your knees (the final position for this movement is with your hands flat on the floor with your thumbs touching, past your feet, and your chin on the lower part of your knee), but don't strain. Keep your back flat and head up until the last moment. Hold and relax in your maximum position for a count of 10. Inhale and return to your seated position stretching your arms above your head. Relax and repeat 3 times.

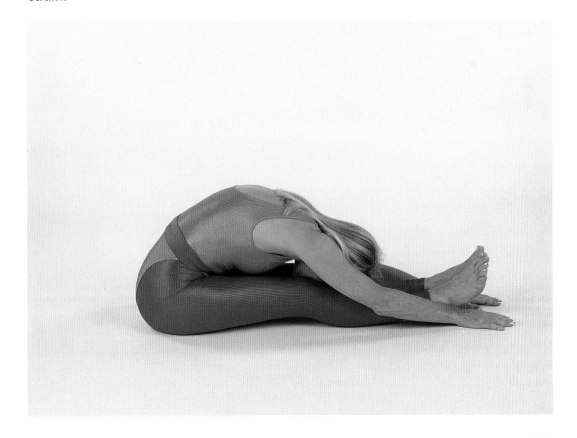

BACK ROLL AND DEEP RELAXATION

Lie flat and lift your knees up to your chest. Interlock your hands together around your knees, and gently rock from one side to the other – one inch to each side is quite sufficient to relax this area. Let your legs go straight out in front of you now and relax.

DEEP RELAXATION

Just allow your body to go completely limp and heavy. Put all thoughts out of your mind. Keep your breathing slow and deep and then, starting with your feet, concentrate on relaxing each muscle in turn, until you have relaxed every muscle in your body.

Now visualise a beautiful peaceful feeling spreading over your body and imagine you are now floating on a lovely blue sea with clear blue sky up above you. Visualise yourself drifting on and on, floating under a beautiful blue sky and relax, relax, relax.

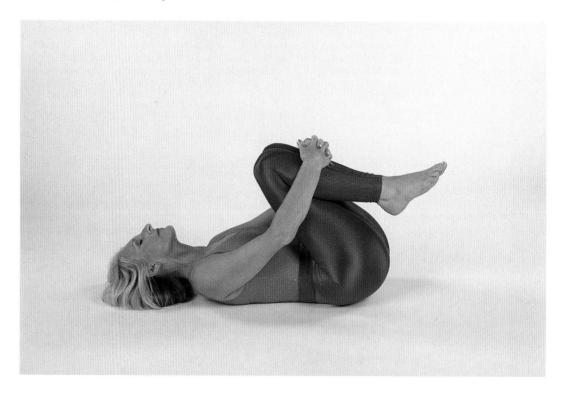

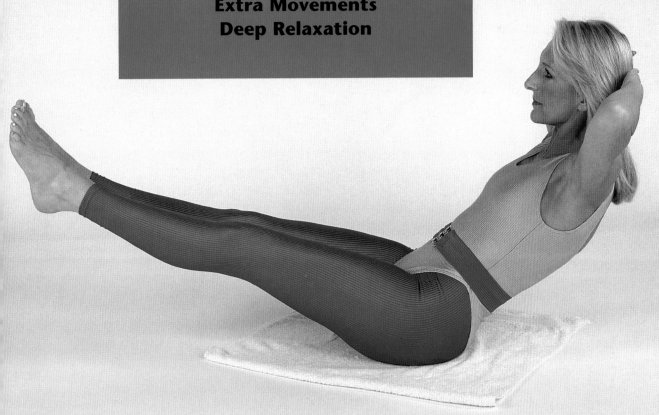

LESSON EIGHT

Energising Deep Breathing
Half Moon Posture
Standing Stick Balance
Sideways Body Raise
Pose of a Dog
Pose of a Boat
Pose of a Sage
Back Stretch
Pose of Tranquillity
Plough with Extra Movements
Pose of a Fish with
Extra Movements
Deep Relaxation

ENERGISING DEEP BREATHING

This is another of my favourite Yoga deep breathing exercises. I do it whenever my energy level is really sinking and it has never let me down yet! It's a great start to the day – especially in the fresh morning air. But do take care – at first, 5 breaths may make you feel a little giddy. If this is the case then start with one breath and build up to 5 slowly.

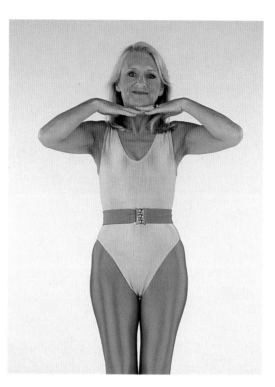

● Stand straight, feet together, and interlock your fingers under your chin, palms down.

● Inhale deeply through your nose for a count of 5. As you do this lift your elbows.

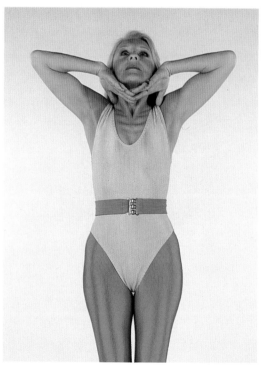

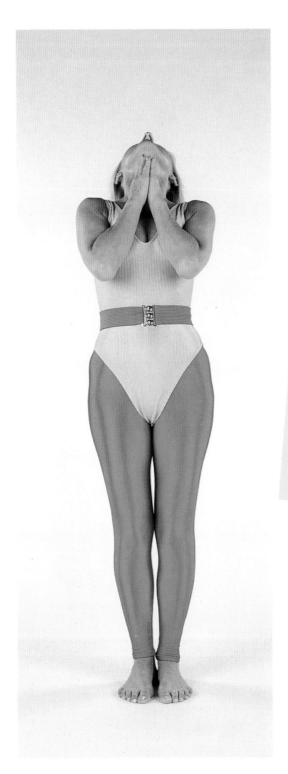

● Drop your head back slightly as you exhale through your mouth, drawing your elbows together. Bring your head up again, draw your elbows up and repeat 5 times.

Although by Yoga standards I am still a beginner, I can feel myself becoming more flexible and my back stronger all the time. To me it has been like a miracle!

M.T.

HALF MOON POSTURE

We first learned this movement in Lesson One (see pp14-15). When you did this in Lesson One you probably found it quite difficult. Keep practicing and it will get easier. Remember, it is excellent for the flexibility of the spine and also for toning the midriff and waistline.

● Stand straight, feet together, with your hands above your head and the inside of your arms, by your ears. The arms straight and together.

● Inhale and as you exhale push your hips to the left and bend to the right, looking forwards. Take care not to twist your body. Hold for a count of 5 then inhale and return to a standing position. Repeat on the other side. Then repeat the whole exercise.

● Return to a standing position and stretch both arms in the air. Inhale and stretch backwards then exhale and breath normally in the movement.

● Inhale and stretch up. Exhale as you stretch forwards and aim your hands by your feet and your head to your knees.

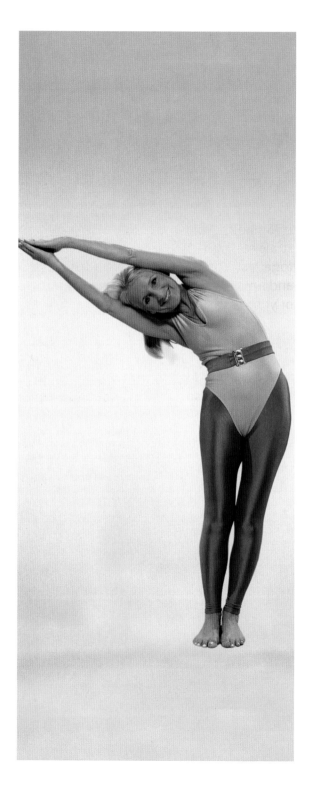

STANDING STICK BALANCE

This beautiful movement firms the hips, thighs and buttocks. It also tones virtually the whole body and is excellent for revving up the circulation.

● Standing straight, place your arms straight above your head, hands together and thumbs crossed. Inhale and place your left foot two feet in front of your right.

● Then, as you exhale, stretch forwards and lift your left leg so that your body forms a capital T, arms and trunk stretched forwards and left leg stretched back. Balance in the movement, starting with a hold for a count of 5 and, as you become more comfortable, gradually increase it to a count of 10, breathing normally. Inhale and return to a standing position. Stretch both arms in the air then gently lower them and repeat on the other side. Repeat on each side.

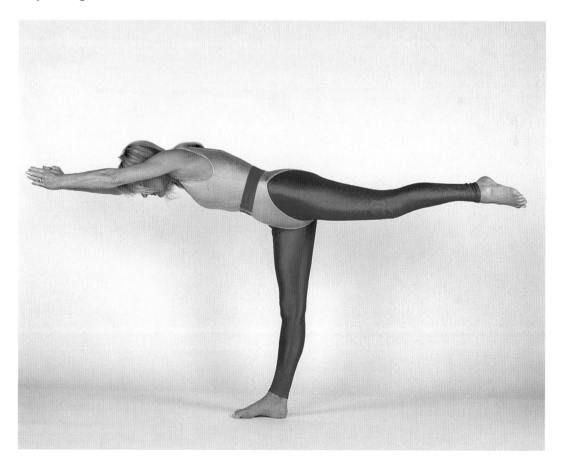

SIDEWAYS BODY RAISE

This is excellent for strengthening the arms and wrists and for making sure they are beautifully toned. But do be careful: to begin with the wrists can be very weak. If you find this exercise difficult, attempt it following the directions but *do not lift your bottom* at first. Wait until the wrists and hands are sufficiently strengthened.

● Place both hands on the floor to the left side of you and lift your body so your weight is on both hands and both feet. Now adjust your body so that your body line is straight, with your shoulder above your wrist. Gently lift your bottom and place your upper foot on the top of the lower. When you feel strong enough, gradually lift your right arm from the floor.

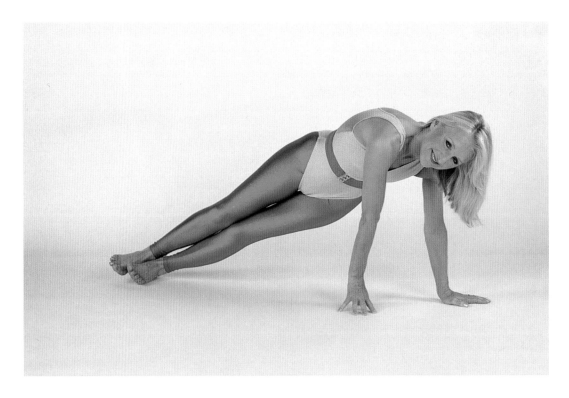

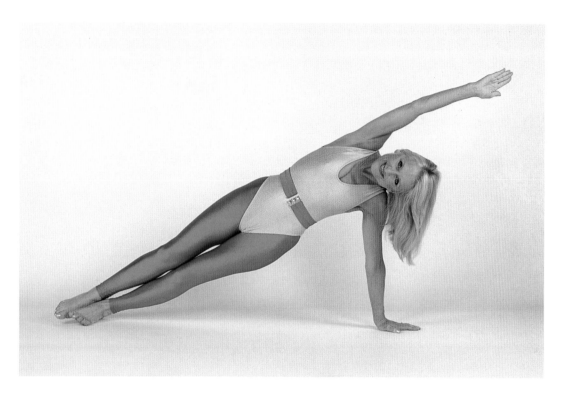

● Make sure your left arm is straight and your right arm is alongside your right ear so your body is perfectly balanced. Concentrate and hold for a count of 5, breathing normally. Then relax, lower your bottom to the floor and repeat on the other side.

Barbara's Yoga classes are super. My back and spine are much more flexible and I hardly ever get backache now. My friends seem to be shrinking while I am standing taller than ever before. It's also a good feeling to be more flexible than your own teenage children!

J.A.F.

POSE OF A DOG

**CAUTION:
DO NOT ATTEMPT IF YOU
ARE PREGNANT**

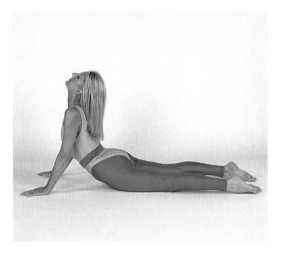

Animals instinctively stretch their spines after a rest to ensure that they are tension free and ready for action. This brilliant movement relieves tension from the lower back, keeps the spine flexible, tones the hands, wrists, thighs and calves and is excellent for ridding the shoulders of stiffness and tension.

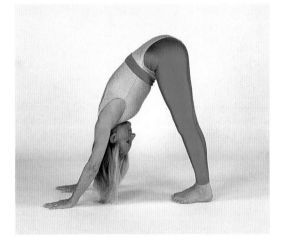

● Lie on your stomach with your legs together and hands just below shoulder level. Inhale and come up into the Cobra position, as in Lesson Three (see pp42-3). Hold for a few seconds, breathing normally.

● Then lift your bottom and drop your head so that your body resembles an inverted V. Stretch your heels down to the floor and draw your head down aiming at your feet. Hold in this position and experience this lovely tension-relieving stretch for 5, then slowly and carefully draw your head forward. Then lower your legs to the floor and gently drop your head back in another Cobra for a count of 5, and lower your body slowly to the floor. Relax and repeat once only.

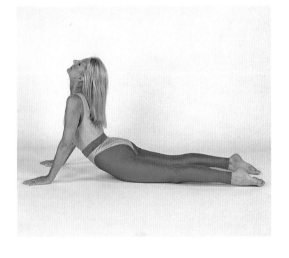

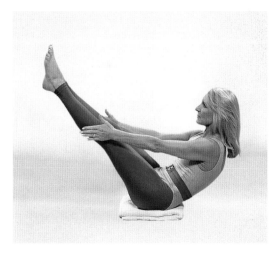

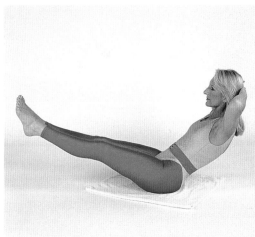

POSE OF A BOAT

**CAUTION:
DO NOT ATTEMPT IF YOU
ARE PREGNANT**

This is hard work, but worth it as it tones the tummy and thighs all in one go and also strengthens the back.

● Sit straight with your legs straight out in front of you and your arms parallel to your legs. Inhale and then exhale and lean back, lifting your legs. Hold for a count of 1 to begin with, gradually increasing to a count of 10 as the muscles get stronger. Remember, *never* strain. Repeat 3 times.

● After you have practiced this movement and feel comfortable with it, try this slightly stronger stretch. Sit with your legs straight out in front of you, placing your hands interlocked behind your head and repeat as above.

● After this movement, lie down, and draw your knees to your chest, interlock your hands around your knees and gently rock from side to side to relax your lower back.

POSE OF A SAGE

This is excellent for relieving tension in the lower back and shoulders. It firms the backs of the thighs and calves and ensures excellent flexibility of the spine.

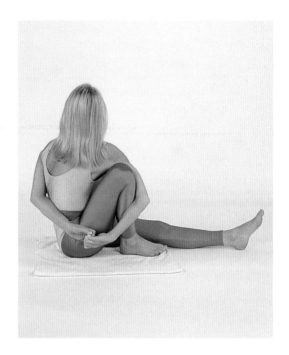

● Sit straight with both legs straight out in front of you. Inhale and bring your right foot by your right buttock. Place your right arm on the inside of your right leg and take it around that leg and behind your back. Take your left hand behind your back and try to join your hands. Don't worry if you can't, just leave them in your maximum position.

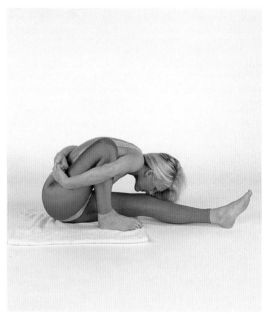

● Inhale and turn your head and torso to the left, then slowly return your head to the front, exhale and, bending gently forwards, aim your chin to your knee. Don't worry, this will take quite a while – *don't strain*. Relax in your maximum movement. Hold for a count of 5, then inhale and return to an upright position, exhale, relax. Repeat to the other side. Repeat once on each side.

BACK STRETCH

This a such an important movement (see p33). It massages the heart, rejuvenates the spine and tones all the abdominal organs. Each time you practice you will manage a little more.

● Sit straight with both legs straight out in front of you, arms stretched in parallel to the legs.

● Breathe in and slowly stretch your arms up as high as possible. Exhale and stretch forwards without strain.

● Clasp your legs and gently lower your chin to your knees. With practice, you will be able to do this – but don't strain, it could take a while. Hold your maximum position for a count of 10. Eventually you will be able to extend both hands past the feet with the thumbs joined and the chin past the knees. Relax and hold this position when accomplished for a count of 10, breathing normally. Breathe in and return to your seated position stretching your arms straight above your head and relax. Repeat 3 times.

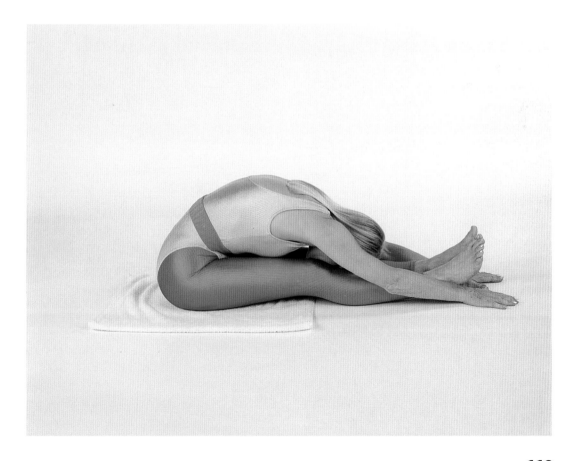

I have always been a couch potato and have never been able to continue in any exercise programme. Every now and again I took up some sport or exercise, only to give it up in a couple of weeks — hating the sweatiness, the agony and total boredom of jogging, aerobics or whatever.

On turning 50, I took a long hard look at my immobile life, my spreading tum and regular visits to the Osteopath, and I tried again. By chance I happened upon Barbara's Yoga classes and I loved them. Six months later I am still attending her class once a week, wake up with Yoga exercises every morning, and intend to go to two classes a week very soon. My mobility has increased amazingly — being able to bend down from a standing position and touch my knees with my nose! — and I have not needed to go to my Osteopath once since I started.

R.R.

I find Yoga very relaxing. After the relaxation session I could easily go to sleep!

R.J.

Yoga has produced a flexibility and suppleness that I thought was lost forever!

W.A.

POSE OF TRANQUILLITY

Caution: Do not attempt this movement if you have high blood pressure or any problem with the head or neck area.

This movement is wonderful for the skin and hair, and also tones the muscles of the spine. It helps to relieve varicose veins, haemorrhoids and aching feet, and is very relaxing.

● Lie flat on your back with your hands relaxed by your sides. Breathe in, then breathe out and slowly lift your legs and buttocks off the floor and gently push yourself up into a high shoulderstand. Allow your knees to drop into the palms of your hands. Keep your elbows straight. Your legs can either be together or apart. Remain in this position for up to 30 seconds at first, increasing at the rate of 30 seconds each month, until you are holding for up to 5 minutes, breathing normally.

● Don't be impatient if you find the balance in this position difficult to obtain at first. It is worth working at and it will soon be the exercise you turn to to help you unwind.

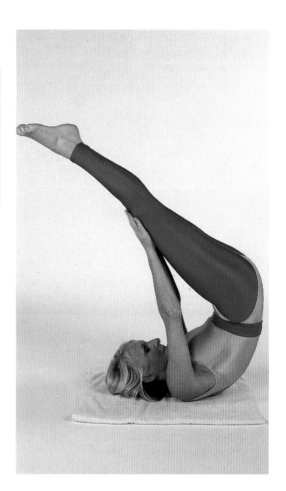

● To come out of this movement, replace your hands by your sides, take your knees to your forehead and very slowly roll down your back, one vertebra at a time. Let both legs go straight out in front of you and relax.

PLOUGH WITH EXTRA MOVEMENTS

Caution: Do not attempt this movement if you have high blood pressure or any problem with the head or neck area.

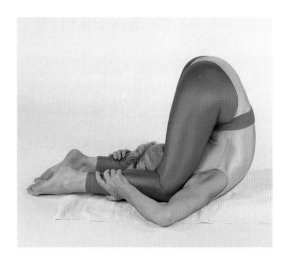

We have practiced the early stages of this movement in Lesson Three (pp48-9) and Four (p66). Now stretch just as far as you can and attempt the stronger stretch *only* when you are ready.

● Lie flat on your back. Breathe in, then exhale and slowly lift both your legs and buttocks off the floor, lifting them as far as you can without strain. If necessary, support your back by placing your hands at your waistline. As your spine becomes more supple, your the feet will touch the floor behind your head and eventually you will be able to bring your knees to the floor by your ears for a really advanced stretch.

● When you are *really* flexible, try to cross your ankles and lift your head for a further advanced stretch – but please remember, this is a *very* strong movement – don't strain.

● To come out of this position, lower your knees to your forehead, and then gently roll, one vertebra at a time,

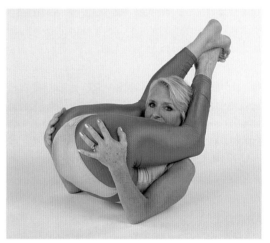

down your back until your bottom touches the floor. Rock the spine gently from side to side, then slowly stretch both legs straight out in front of you and relax.

122

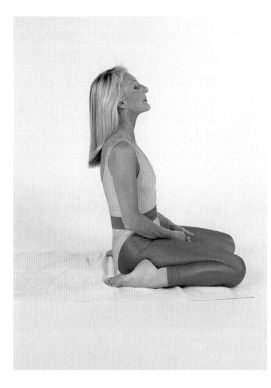

POSE OF A FISH WITH EXTRA MOVEMENTS

We first tried the Fish in Lesson Six (see p94). It is excellent for the throat and neck, it also helps expand the chest and relieve tightness in it and can be a great help for asthmatics. When and *only when* you are comfortable with the Fish you may try this stronger variation, which is excellent for slimming the thighs, firming the abdomen and increasing flexibility in the knees, ankles and hips.

● Kneel with your bottom on your heels, knees 1 foot apart (or a little more), then with your hands on the floor either side of you, try to lower your bottom between your heels. For some this is easy; if so proceed. If there is any pull at all, just practice this each day but go no further until you can comfortably sit between your heels. It might take a while, but cheer up – you will regain your flexibility.

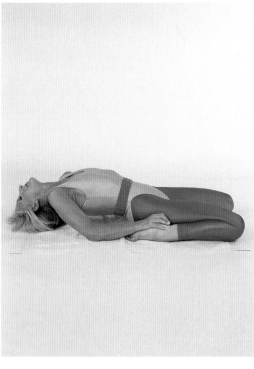

● With your bottom on the floor between your heels, place your hands on your feet, lift your head and place the top of your head on the floor. Hold for a count of 5 to begin with and, when it becomes really comfortable, take 5 big deep breaths in the pose, exhaling slowly after each one. Then inhale, return to a kneeling position and then lie flat on the floor and relax.

123

DEEP RELAXATION: HOW TO RE-ENERGISE

Lie flat and relax each muscle in turn. Keep your breathing slow and deep. Feel yourself becoming very calm and relaxed. Roll your eyeballs upwards, let your eyelids become heavy and feel your body sinking into the floor. Now visualise a beautiful lake surrounded by lovely trees of many shades of green and see the surface of the lake ruffled by the breeze. Breathe slowly and deeply and watch as the lake surface becomes smooth and as it does so feel your tensions floating away.

Now the lake is calm and peaceful, visualise the sun coming out making the water sparkle. As the sun comes out see the lovely sunlight and watch the lake surface sparkle. As you visualise this feel new energy flowing into your body dispelling tiredness and filling you with new life, energy and sparkle. Keep this in your mind for 5-10 minutes then take a deep breath and stretch and have a great day.

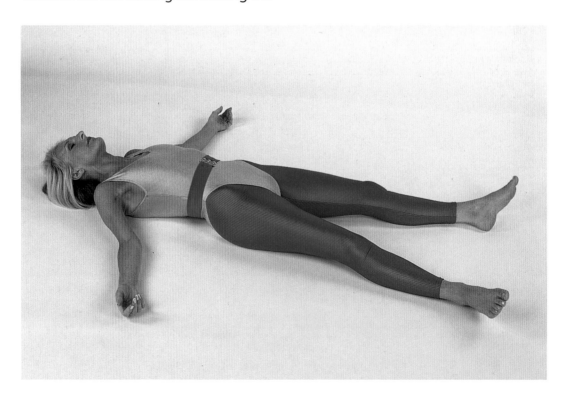

LESSON NINE

Start your day with the beautiful Salute to the Sun sequence from Lesson Five (see pages 68-72).

Half Moon Balance
Toe Balance
Pose of a Heron
Spinal Stretch
Wide-Angled Leg Stretch
Pose of a Plane
Camel and Diamond Position
Pose of a Rabbit
Shoulderstand and Cycle
Pose of a Fish
Relaxation

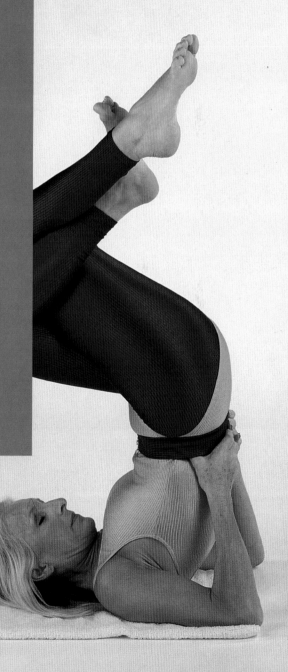

HALF MOON BALANCE

This movement is excellent for increasing the flexibility of the hip joints and lower back and for toning and slimming the hips and thighs.

● Stand straight, inhale and place your right hand out to the side. Now lean over and place it on the floor (bend your knees if you need to).

● Now exhale and lift your left leg out to the side and your left arm straight up in the air. Gently open out the chest and carefully turn your head to look at the ceiling. Hold at first for a count of 5, but increase to 10 with practice. Inhale and return to a standing position. Repeat on the other side and then repeat once on both sides.

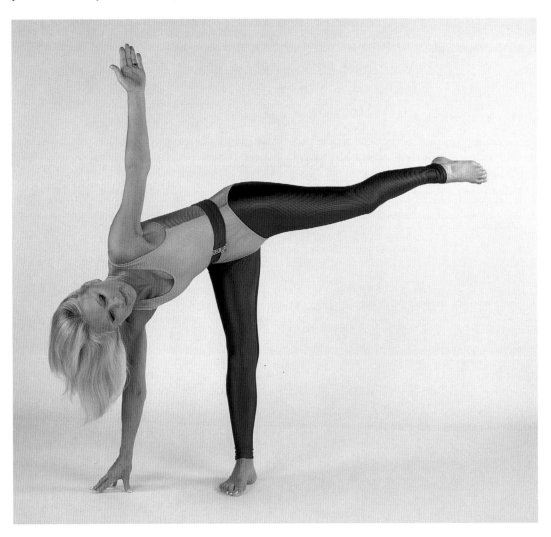

TOE BALANCE

As soon as – and not *until* – you feel comfortable with the Awkward Posture (see p29) you may like to try the Toe Balance. This one is particularly brilliant for toning and keeping flexible all the muscles in the legs and feet. The balances are also wonderful for helping you concentrate and giving you a lovely sense of calm and peace.

● With your feet 1 foot apart, squat down on your toes, placing your left hand on the floor. Concentrate on a spot to help you balance.

● Pick up your right big toe in your right hand and gradually straighten your leg. When you are comfortably balanced, place your left hand on your left knee and hold for a count of 5, then gently lower your leg and relax. Repeat on the other side.

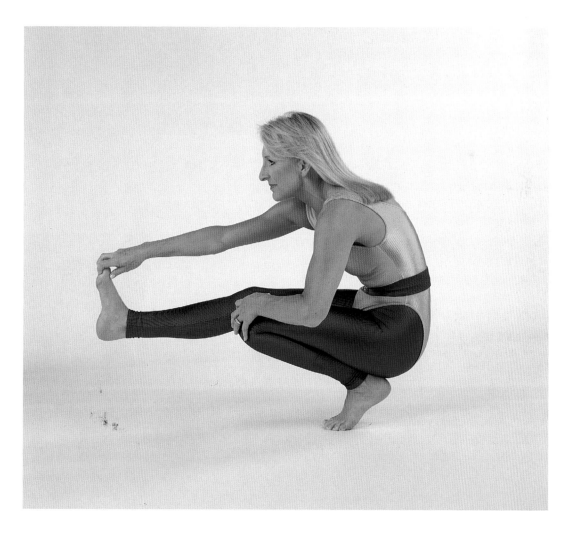

POSE OF A HERON

This movement tones the backs of the thighs, stretches the hamstrings and firms the buttocks. It is excellent for helping to remove cellulite from the backs of the thighs. Think of how slim a heron's thighs are – no cellulite there! Believe me, this exercise is worth it, so do practice it as often as possible without strain.

Stage One
● Sit straight and, bending your left knee, bring your left foot into the middle between your legs.

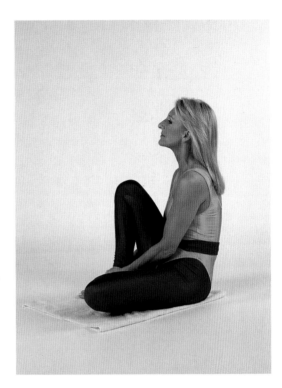

● Inhale and clasp your hands under your right foot. Keeping your back straight exhale and gently straighten your right leg, drawing your knee to your nose or your maximum position in this movement (if you can't manage to straighten your leg while holding your foot, simply clasp your calf instead). Hold for a count of 5, then gently lower your leg. Repeat on the other side, then repeat on both sides.

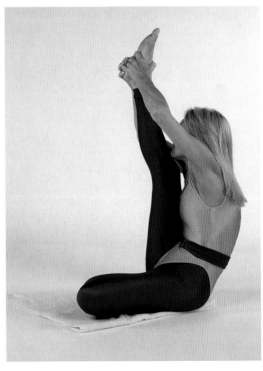

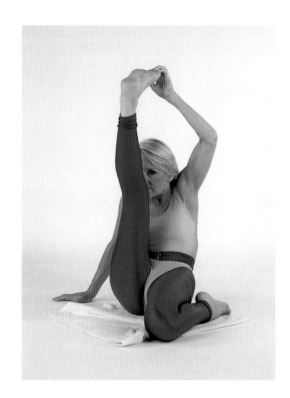

Stage Two

When you are comfortable with Pose of a Heron Stage One, try Stage Two for a slightly stronger stretch.

● Place your left foot carefully by your left buttock and take your right foot in your left hand, placing your right hand on the floor for support. Inhale and gently try to straighten your right leg, drawing it towards your nose as you exhale. When you no longer need your right hand for support, try to clasp your right foot with both hands. Hold for a count of 5, then gently lower your leg, relax and repeat to the other side.

For many years I had been unsupple and was getting worse. For instance, to touch my toes was out of the question and even putting on my socks was difficult. After 18 months of Yoga, once a week, I can now touch my toes with ease and many other movements are much easier.

I feel that I am getting more supple as I get older which can't be bad!

B.S.

SPINAL STRETCH

This movement is excellent for your balance and concentration. It is also brilliant for firming and toning all the muscles in the legs. Normally as we get older our bottom drops and our thighs lose their smoothness. This stretch keeps the hamstrings in excellent condition and the lumps and bumps just float away.

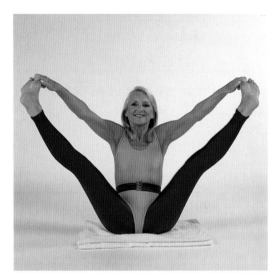

● Make sure your blanket is thick enough to cushion your bottom. Bring both feet into the middle and grab your big toes. Inhale, focus on a spot in front of you and then gradually exhale and lift your legs from the floor. (When we first start this we all get a fit of giggles and wobbles, but it *is* possible. Go slowly and don't worry if you can't straighten your legs at first. Just concentrate and practice and it will happen.) Gradually straighten your legs. Hold for a count of 5, breathing normally, then gently lower your legs to the floor and relax. As you practice this movement you will gain amazing control.

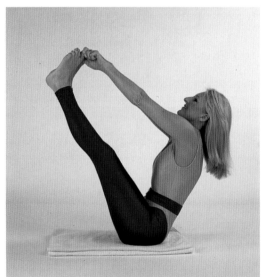

● For an advanced stretch, try to draw your feet together while balanced! You can actually feel this firming the thighs! Repeat once.

WIDE–ANGLED LEG STRETCH

Further movements for this lovely exercise that we started in Lesson Four (see pp64-5). Now, for a really flexible back and thighs, try to move just a little further – but *never* strain.

● Sit straight with both legs very wide apart, both arms parallel to your right leg.

● Breathe in, then breathe out and slowly lean forwards, clasping the furthest part of your leg and take your chin towards your right knee. (Eventually you will clasp your feet and take your head to your knee, but this will only come with practice.) Relax in this position for a count of 5, breathing normally, then slowly lift your head, breathe in and slowly come up into a sitting position. Repeat to the other side.

● Now place your hands on your knees. Breathe in and as you exhale, slowly slide your hands towards your toes. Then, with your back flat and your head up, slowly take your chin towards the floor. Relax in your maximum position in this movement (eventually your chin will reach the floor), hold for a count of 10 and then slowly lift your head. Breathe in, return to a sitting position and relax. Repeat this movement 3 times.

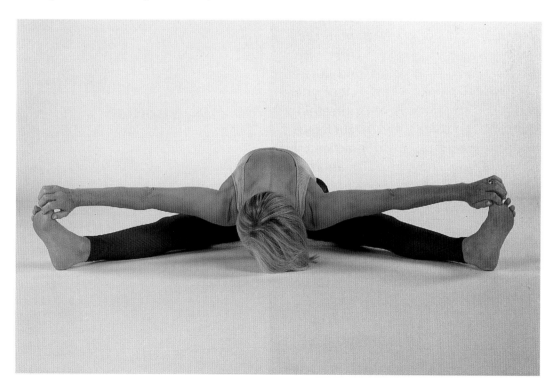

POSE OF A PLANE

This great movement strengthens the arms and wrists and removes tension from the shoulders. It is also is excellent for the flexibility of the hips and lower back.

● Sit on the floor with both legs stretched straight out in front of you and place your hands on the floor comfortably behind your back, fingers pointing backwards.

Stage One
● Inhale and as you exhale lift your body from the floor, keeping your feet and toes on the floor. With your body in a lovely straight line, let your head drop back and hold for a count of 5, then gently lower your body to the floor. Repeat.

Stage Two
● When you feel comfortable in the movement lift your body from the floor as in Stage One, then lift your right leg and point your toes upwards. Hold the movement for a count of 1, then lower your leg and lift the other one, hold and lower. Then lower your body down to the floor and relax.

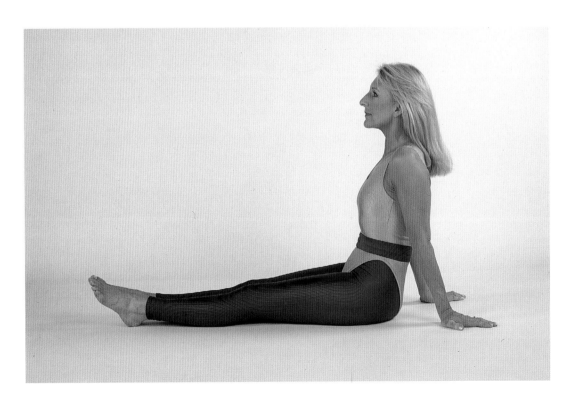

Stage One

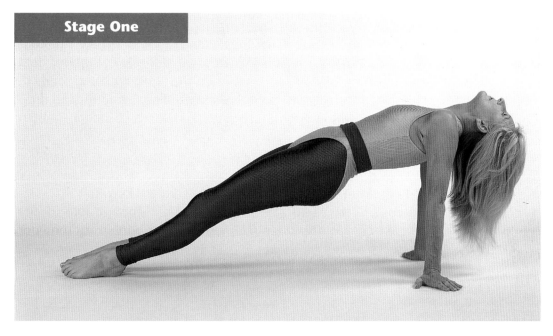

Stage Two

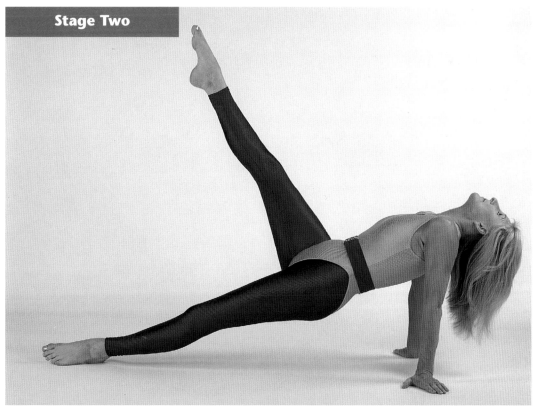

CAMEL AND DIAMOND POSITION

We have practiced the Camel in Lesson Two (see pp 30-31). Here we will repeat it and try an extra stretch.

● Adopt a high kneeling position with your hands at your waistline, thumbs in front and fingers behind, knees and feet 1 foot apart. Breathe in deeply and allow your upper body to bend backwards, keeping your thighs straight. Exhale once you have reached your maximum position. If you can, place your right hand on your right foot and your left hand on your left foot. Breathe normally in your maximum position and hold for 5 seconds. Inhale as your return to an upright position.

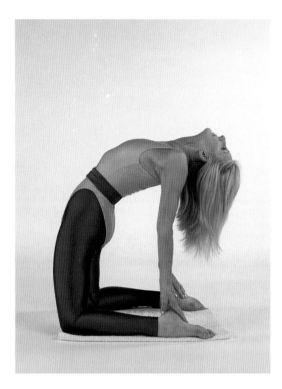

● Exhale and allow your bottom to sink to your heels with your hands by your sides and your head on the floor in front of you and relax in the Pose of a Child.

DIAMOND POSITION

Once your body becomes really flexible, from your maximum Camel position try the Diamond Position where, bending your elbows, you eventually take your head to the floor. (Go carefully until your body becomes really flexible. Always make sure that you progress safely and that for every inch you lower your body towards the floor you can easily bring yourself up again.) This gives a brilliant stretch to the thighs and

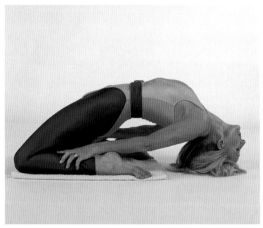

spine. Hold your maximum position for a count of 5, then inhale and return to an upright position. Exhale and relax in the Pose of a Child.

134

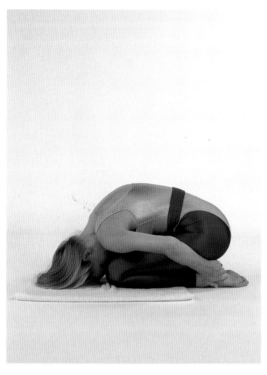

POSE OF A RABBIT

Caution: Do not attempt this movement if you have high blood pressure or any problem with the head or neck area.

This movement is excellent for releasing tension from the neck and can be most helpful for headache sufferers. Due to increase in blood circulation, it is wonderful for the skin and hair, it tones the thyroid, parathyroid glands and stimulates blood to the pituitary gland and the pineal body.

● Kneel on your mat or towel and place your forehead on the front of your knees, your hands on the soles of your feet.

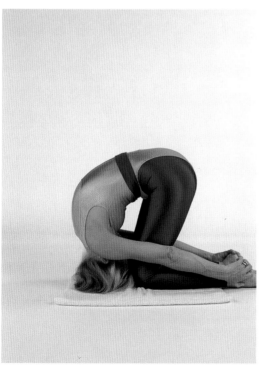

● Inhale and as you exhale gently start to lift your bottom from your heels. Your aim is to have your bottom pointing to the ceiling, but remember, go at your own pace, without strain. Hold in your maximum position for a count of 5, increasing to 10 as you gain confidence in this movement. Then gently lower your bottom to your heels and relax. Do not lift your head immediately, count to 10 slowly. Then return to a kneeling position and relax. Do not repeat.

SHOULDERSTAND

Caution: Do not attempt this movement if you have high blood pressure or any problem with the head or neck area.

We started this movement in Lesson Six (see pp92-3). Now we will continue and, if you are ready, we will start to do the magical Shoulderstand Cycle.

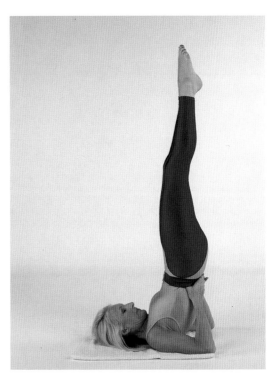

● Lie flat with your hands relaxed by your sides, palms down. Breathe in deeply, then exhale and slowly lift your legs and buttocks off the floor. Keep lifting them until you reach your maximum position, supporting your back by placing your hands at your waistline.

● To come out of this movement, draw your knees to your forehead and roll down your back one vertebra at a time. Interlock your hands around your knees, rock your back from side to side and relax. Once mastered, you may try the movements in the cycle. Please try only one at a time before doing all three.

SHOULDERSTAND AND EAGLE BALANCE: For really flexible legs, hips and knees. Support your back in the Shoulderstand, then carefully wind the left leg around the right as in the Eagle Balance Standing. Unwind and repeat on the other side.

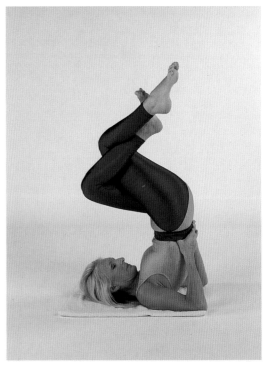

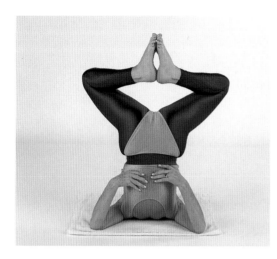

SHOULDERSTAND AND PAGODA:

This is excellent for your waist and the flexibility of your hips. Support your back with both hands, open your legs wide, then place the soles of your feet together. Carefully twist the body to the right. Slowly return, then repeat to the other side. Gently stretch your legs back into the Shoulderstand again.

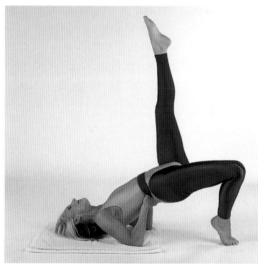

SHOULDERSTAND AND THE BRIDGE:

This is excellent for improving both the flexibility and strength of the spine. Support your back with both hands and gently try to drop 1 foot to touch the floor. Keeping your back arched, lift the foot up again and repeat on the other side.

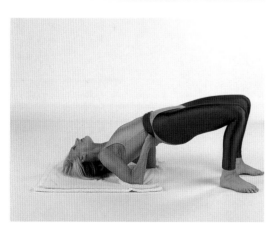

● Then, making sure that your arms are fully supporting the weight of your lower body, try to drop both feet, one at a time, into the Bridge position. Then try to lift both legs up again one at a time – but remember do it carefully and gently and *without strain*. If you manage the Bridge but can't get up again, simply lower your back to the floor and relax. Keep trying, you will be able to do it eventually.

POSE OF A FISH

● Following the Shoulderstand, lie flat, arch your upper body, place your hands under your buttocks and the top of your head on the floor. Hold for a count of 10, breathing slowly and deeply in the movement. Then come out of the movement, lie flat and relax.

RELAXATION

Lie flat on your back with your hands palms uppermost. Slow down your breathing and consciously relax each muscle in turn. Roll your eyeballs upwards and let your eyelids become heavy and feel your whole body becoming increasingly comfortable. Now imagine you are in a beautiful wood with really tall trees around you, soft green moss and ferns abound. Visualise the sunlight filtering through these lovely trees giving a golden light to everything it touches. Imagine the lovely fresh scent of the pine trees and listen to the birds singing. Now keep this in your mind and relax, relax, relax.

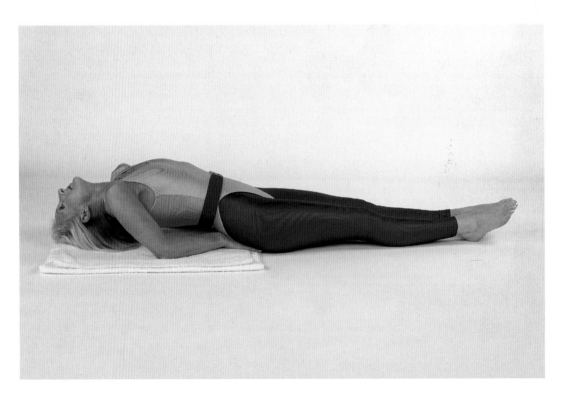

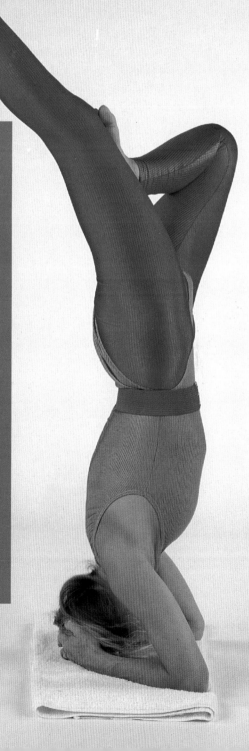

LESSON TEN

WHEEL

Yoga's ultimate backwards stretch. We previously practiced this movement in Lesson Seven (p104-5) I am repeating it for your convenience. It is great for energising the entire body and keeping your spine flexible for life.

● Lie flat on the floor and place both hands by your ears, fingers pointing to your shoulders. Place your feet flat on the floor, about 1 foot apart. Inhale and as you exhale lift your body and rest your head on the floor. Hold, then gently lower your body to the floor. Draw your knees to your chest and gently rock your back from side to side. When you have managed this stage comfortably, try the Wheel.

● Lie on the floor, hands by your ears and palms flat, with your fingers pointing to your shoulders, feet about 1 foot apart and knees bent. Inhale deeply and as you exhale lift your entire body from the floor.

● Eventually try to straighten your arms and legs and push as high as possible. Then, breathing normally in the position try to hold it for a count of 5. Lengthening your hold as you progress in the movement.

● Gently lower your body to the floor, draw your knees to your chest, and rock from side to side. Lie flat and relax.

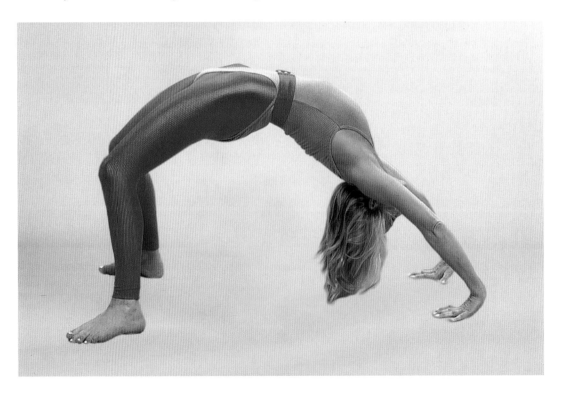

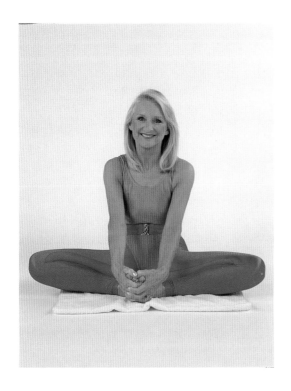

THIGH STRETCH AND STAR

We first practiced this in Lesson Five (see p79). This movement tones the inner thighs and keeps the hip joints really supple. It is excellent for the pelvic floor and is beneficial for both men and women for the health of the urinary system.

● Sit very straight and bring both feet towards your body, placing the soles of your feet together and clasping them in both hands. Breathe in, then breathe out. Gently lower your knees to the floor. Hold your maximum position for a count of 5, breathing normally, then slowly return your knees to their upright position and relax. Repeat 3 times.

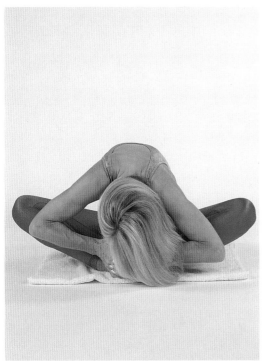

THE STAR: This is excellent for your hips and lower back.

● When the Thigh Stretch movement becomes easy, as you lower your knees to the floor gently draw your chin towards your feet. Hold for a count of 5, relaxing in the movement, and then slowly return to an upright position as you inhale and relax.

LOTUS POSITION AND SCALES

● Sit in a Lotus position (for full instructions see p80). To warm up and loosen your legs for this position, do remember to do the Alternate Leg Pull (see p47) as well as the Thigh Stretch.

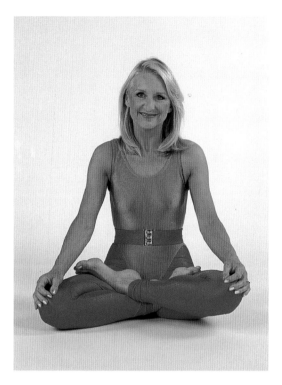

● Place your hands on the floor by your buttocks, inhale deeply and as you exhale gently lift your bottom from the floor. Hold for just a few seconds then lower your body gently and relax.

Congratulations – this is a wonderful achievement. It means that now your hips, ankles and feet really are flexible, and by doing the Scales you are also toning your hands, wrists and arms.

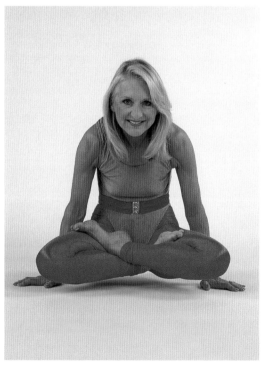

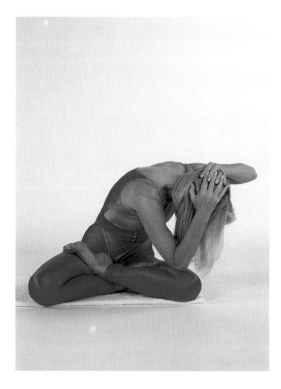

LOTUS POSITION AND TWIST

This movement may be done in either the Full Lotus position, Half Lotus position, or a cross-legged position. The aim is to slim the midriff, waistline and abdomen. It is also marvellous for keeping the spine flexible and able to cope with the knocks and jolts it gets in our everyday life.

Stage One

● Sitting in one of the above positions, interlock your hands behind your head, take a deep breath in and slowly exhale and take your right elbow to your left knee and look behind you. Hold for a count of 5, then breathe in and slowly come up into your sitting position and repeat to the other side. Perform this part of the movement 3 times on each side.

Stage Two

● With your hands interlocked behind your head, exhale deeply and slowly bend forwards, aiming your head towards the floor. Relax in your maximum position and hold, breathing normally, for a count of 5. Breathe in and slowly return to a sitting position. Breathe out and relax and repeat twice.

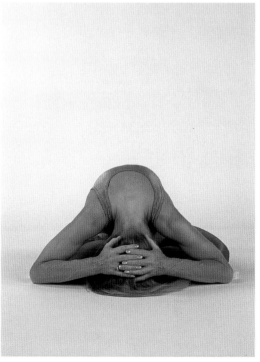

POSE OF A TORTOISE

This is one of Yoga's all time greats! It gives you the most wonderful feeling of calm and peace. It tones all the abdominal organs and releases tension from the spine. It makes you feel refreshed and keeps your hips in perfect condition. Once you have mastered this brilliant stretch you just feel forever young!

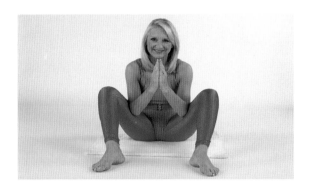

● Sit with your knees bent, about 2 feet apart with feet facing outwards. Inhale and place your hands together. Exhale and, dropping your elbows towards the floor, open your arms and try to place your elbows under your knees. If your elbows do not as yet go under your knees don't worry, persevere and they soon will.

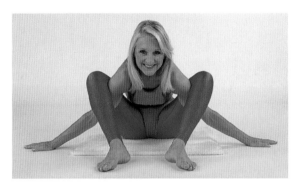

● Inhale, stretch out your arms and then, if your elbows are on the outer side of your knees, stretch out both legs and arms and aim your chin to the floor. Be careful not to strain, and proceed no further until you are able to do this stage. Remain in your maximum position for a count of 10 breathing normally. Then inhale and, drawing your feet in first, gradually return to a sitting position.

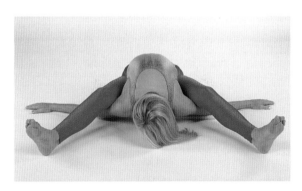

● After you have mastered this movement, try the next stage. In your maximum position, take your hands behind your back and try to interlock them.

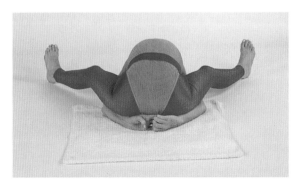

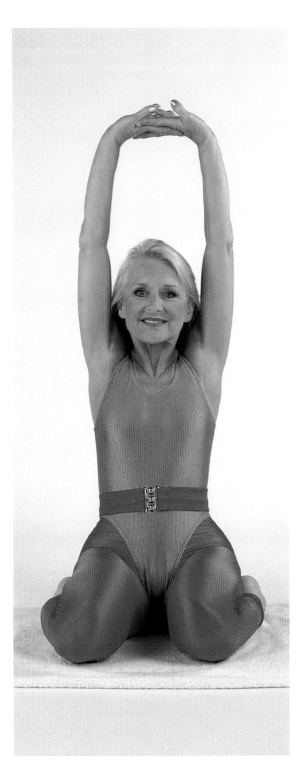

POSE OF A MOUNTAIN

This is brilliant for the shoulders and the arms – we really do shoulder our problems and this beautiful movement acts like magic in relieving the pressure from our shoulders and re-aligning them. It's ideal if you are leaning over a computer or on the phone all day.

● Sit in a kneeling position and interlock your fingers together. Inhale and, inverting your hands, stretch your arms up above your head. Bring them back so the insides of your arms are in line with your ears. Hold, breathing normally, for a few seconds then undo your arms and slowly lower them.

● When and if your knees are sufficiently flexible, a stronger move in this position is when the buttocks are on the floor between your heels. *Never* strain however, this will come with practice. (To help you lower your bottom in between your heels, kneel with your feet about 1 foot apart, place your hands on your feet and very carefully lower your bottom onto the floor keeping your body's weight on your hands.)

I first started to experience back pain when pregnant with my second child, at 34. Over the next 15 years I was regularly treated by osteopaths and would gain relief for short periods, but always the back pain would return. In 1994, I was working at an exhibition when I came out in a rash all over my body and this was diagnosed as being the result of stress. At the same time a friend had started yoga lessons with Barbara and was already feeling the benefits, so I thought there was nothing to lose!

I have now been practicing Yoga regularly for 3 years and the back pain has all but disappeared. If I ever get even a twinge I feel cheated. Also, I feel far less stressed and my whole outlook is more relaxed.

Now, I can't imagine my life without Yoga.

N.C.

When feeling tired, depressed, at odds with one-and-all, an hour spent at Barbara's Yoga workout suddenly makes you feel that you can cope; the energy is there to face the world with a smile on your face!

J.K.

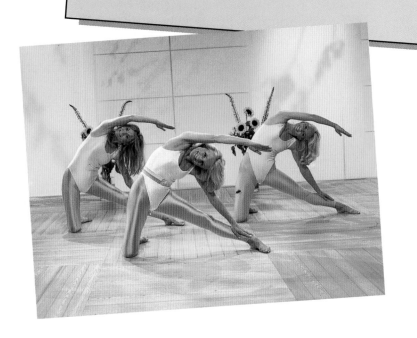

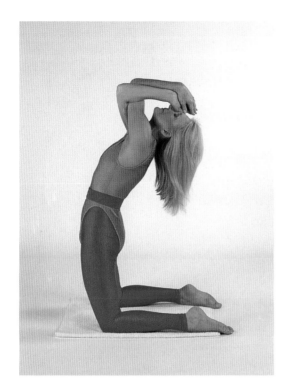

HEAD OF A HORSE EXERCISES

This is one of my favourite movements. It lifts the bust, firms the upper arms, gets rid of tension in the neck and firms the jaw.

Stage One

● In a high kneeling position, place your arms straight out in front of you, cross the left upper arm over the right and take that arm under it, so the palms of the hands are together. Now place the first joint of your thumb in the hollow above your nose and inhale. Then, with a full lung, bend backwards to your own maximum position without strain. Exhale, then hold for a count of 8, breathing normally. Inhale and return to an upright position, then relax. Then repeat on the opposite side.

Stage Two

This movement has the extra benefits of aiding the flexibility of the knees, ankles and hips and is a great toner for the upper and inner thigh – but remember, don't strain.

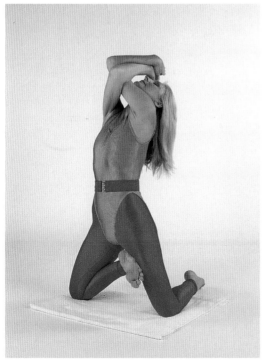

Come into an all fours position and then carefully try to place your right foot on your left thigh, keeping your right knee on the floor. Then come up into a high kneeling position, keeping your right foot on your thigh. For the arm movement, proceed as Stage One and reverse the legs and arms to do the other side.

147

CLASSICAL HEADSTAND

Please do not attempt this movement until you have achieved all the other exercises with comfort, as by then your body will have improved in both flexibility and strength.

However, you must never attempt this movement if you have high blood pressure, have had a neck injury or have any problems with the eyes or ears. Please do not do this movement if you are suffering from catarrh or sinusitis or have any problems with the head or neck area.

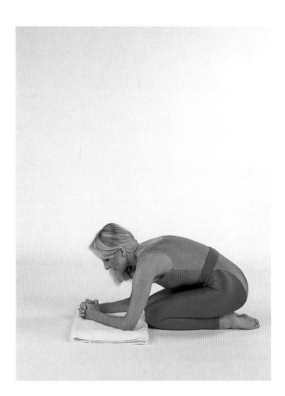

This is one of Yoga's greatest exercises. It is wonderfully refreshing and invigorating. It firms the abdominal muscles, is marvellous for the skin and hair, and can help insomnia if performed at night before bed. In the *Hatha Yoga Pradipika* it states 'do the headstand daily and in six months grey hair and wrinkles completely disappear' (80-82). If you would like to try this movement, do proceed with caution.

● Kneel and place your hands interlocked together on the floor. Lift one hand and place it at the centre of the other elbow. This ensures you have the elbows the correct distance apart, then re-interlock your hands. Place your head in the cup formed by your hands.

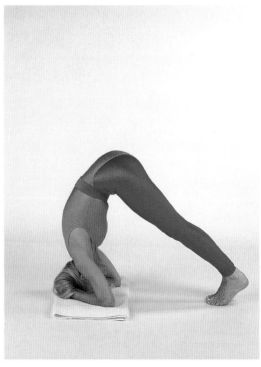

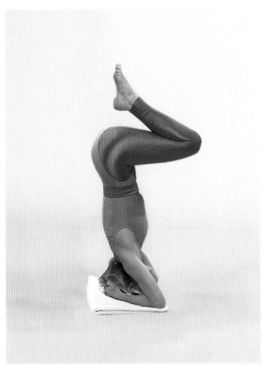

● Lift your bottom in the air and walk your feet in towards your head. Practice these two movements every day for two weeks and you may then progress to the next stage. (This is very important as it is vital that your head and neck area are accustomed to being in an inverted position before you go any further.)

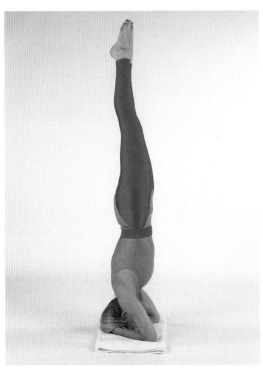

● Lift your feet off the floor into a crouching position and then *gently* straighten your legs. Practice by a wall at first with a soft rug or towel on the floor. Remain in the position as long as is comfortable. Start with just a few seconds, and gradually – over a period of months – increase to 2 minutes. Bend your knees into a crouching position, lower your legs to the floor and then keep your head down for a count of 10 to allow your circulation to return to normal. The headstand is often referred to as the King of all Yoga exercises. Extra blood is drawn to the cells of the brain and this has an incredibly rejuvenating effect on both the mind and body. It gives the student an immediate feeling of energy, vitality and positive health.

CLASSICAL HEADSTAND CYCLE

Once you have gained confidence in the Headstand, try one of these movements at a time before attempting them in sequence as the Headstand Cycle.

EAGLE BALANCE: Assume the Headstand and then entwine one leg around the other, as in the Eagle Standing. Then repeat with the other leg.

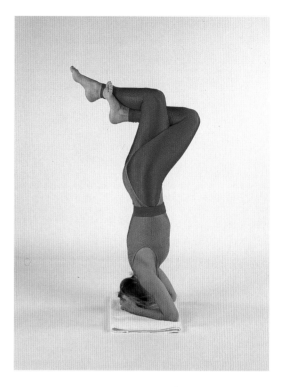

PAGODA: In the Headstand, open your legs wide, place the soles of your feet together and turn your body to the right and then the left.

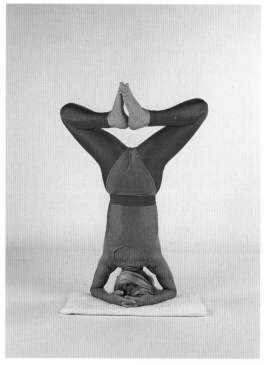

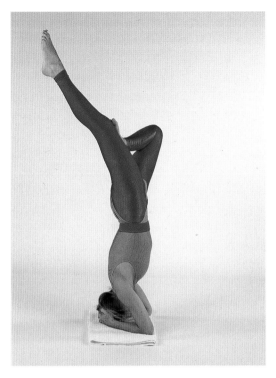

HALF SPLIT: In the Headstand, with your legs together slide one foot slowly down to the other thigh. Return to a full Headstand, then repeat on the other side.

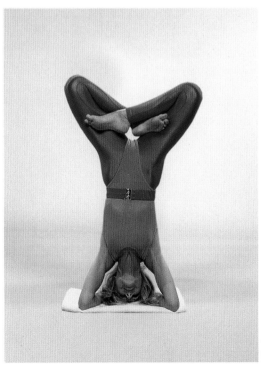

LOTUS: This is only possible when the Full Lotus position becomes comfortable. In the Headstand, gently assume the Lotus position. (This is not easy but it is a great achievement when you make it.)

Well done! This is it! It reverses gravity and does wonders for skin, hair, brain, eyes and ears. It is our elixir of youth.

POSE OF TRANQUILLITY AND FISH IN LOTUS POSITION

Caution: Do not attempt this movement if you have high blood pressure or any problem with the head or neck area.

We first practiced the Pose of Tranquillity in Lesson Eight (see p121). Please refer back to it for the full instructions, and if you are not able to do the Lotus Position, repeat the Pose of Tranquillity as shown there.

● Once you have managed the Lotus Position simply move into it then place your hands by your sides and lie flat and lift your lower body from the floor, supporting your back with your hands. Then take your hands to your knees and again relax in the movement breathing normally.

● To come out of the movement roll slowly down your back until your lower body touches the floor. Then, keeping your legs in Lotus Position, place your hands under your buttocks and arch your back until the top of your head touches the floor in the Pose of a Fish in the Lotus Position. Rest for 1 minute in this position and you'll look and feel so refreshed – it's like a tonic.

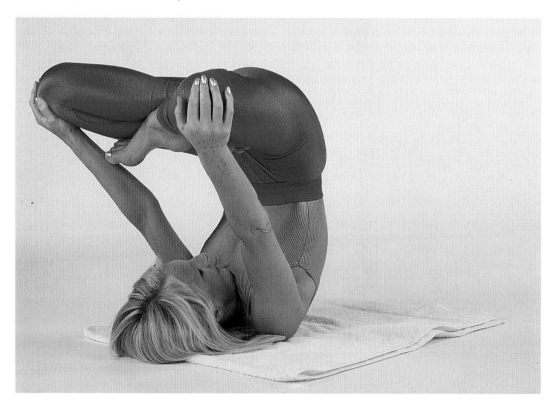

POSE OF A FISH

If you have not yet managed to do the Lotus position. Don't worry. Stick with the simple Fish position.

● Place both legs straight out in front of you and place your hands under your buttocks and arch your back and place the top of your head on the floor.

● Stay in this position, breathing normally, then lower your body to the floor and relax.

RELAXATION

Once again lie flat on your back, palms uppermost and gently relax each muscle in turn. Feel yourself relaxing totally. Let your eyelids become heavy, roll your eyeballs upwards and slow down your breathing and concentrate on exhaling slowly after each breath.

Now with the body really relaxed visualise the most beautiful rainbow you have ever seen. See a wonderful arch of colour in the sky and relax, relax and relax. Let your body relax gently for 5-10 minutes, then gently stretch your body and have a wonderful day.

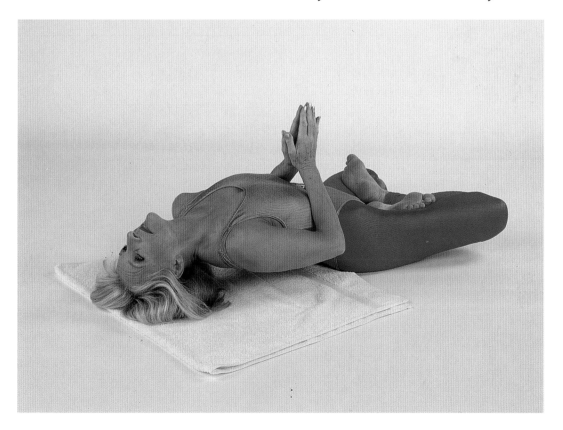

FACIAL EXERCISES

These are my favourite facial exercises. They do look dreadful so make sure you are alone when you do them!

After all the exertion of Lessons One to Ten, it's nice to be able to do something on your sofa - enjoy!

To Firm a Double Chin

This is simple, easy to remember and it works! Sit straight and grin. Then, still grinning very wide, gently drop your head back and open and close your mouth five times. Try to do this 3 times a day.

To Firm the Middle Part of the Neck

If it is just the middle part of your neck that has gone saggy, this really tones the underside of your throat. Sit straight and aim your bottom set of teeth to your nose. Hold for a count of 10 and relax. Repeat 3 times daily.

To Soften Tramlines across the Forehead

This is also blissfully relaxing, very effective and really soothing. Do it anywhere, anytime. Sit straight, close your eyes and place your fingertips touching on the centre of your forehead. Breathe in, then slowly exhale and gently draw your scalp back and lower your eyebrows, and at the same time slowly draw your fingers across your forehead to your hairline. Repeat 5 times.

To Lift the Cheeks

This livens the face, tightens the muscles, stimulates the skin and gives a lovely expression. Sit straight and open your eyes wide. Stretch your upper lip over your teeth and lift the corners of your mouth into a clown-like grin. Hold for a count of 10. Repeat 3 times and do this at least 5 times daily.

Eye Exercises

Your eyes are designed to move in many directions and to react to all light intensities. But now, due to modern technology, we frequently find ourselves in artificial lighting looking at static horizons such as the computer screen. Deep breathing in the fresh air is most beneficial to the eyes, as are a wide variety of light intensities. The following exercises are extremely helpful to the muscles of the eyes.

Sit in a comfortable, cross-legged position and imagine a large clock in front of you. Look upwards at 12 o'clock, then at five past, and continue around the clock, holding each position for a count of 3. Do not strain, at first some of the moves may be a little difficult. Continue round the clock and then repeat in the opposite direction.

Blink two or three times, then rub the palms of your hands together to create warmth and place the warm hands over your closed eyes. This is known as palming the eyes, and is really refreshing for tired or strained eyes.

Scalp Exercise

Have you noticed how much your hair reflects your health? It is often the first part of us to show signs of stress, poor lifestyle or ill health. This scalp exercise is excellent for restoring that healthy sheen. Sit in a comfortable position and place both hands in your hair, fingers spread out. Gently pull your hair, and as you pull it, carefully move your scalp. Continue with other areas of your head until the whole head has been worked. Follow this with an inverted posture to stimulate blood circulation to the hair follicles.

YOGA AND WEIGHT LOSS

One of the most common questions I am asked is 'how will I lose weight with Yoga, if Yoga exercises do not burn fat?' The answer to this is really in your diet. I feel there is little point in burning fat only to continue to eat too many high calorie foods. Once you start Yoga it will help you to lose weight by:

● stimulating your glands to help improve your metabolism
● creating lean muscles which are beautiful, lighter and leaner, which weigh less and look slimmer than those made by muscle-building exercises

● as you get rid of tension you will not be tempted to eat to relieve stress

● as your energy improves you will live more energetically and do more, and food will start to take a more normal role in your day. You will no longer look to food to stimulate your energy and relieve boredom

● your taste buds will naturally change and you will start to lean more towards fresh, natural, healthy foods

● your body will become like a perfectly toned machine; your natural appestat will start to work again so that you will eat no more than is necessary.

Having said that, many of my pupils have asked me to guide them, so in the following pages you will find a healthy meal plan that they have tried and tested for you.

I changed my own diet thirty-five years ago to natural foods. The result was amazing. I lost weight but, more than that, I looked and felt better than I had done for ages. My skin looked better and my energy level soared. Thirty-five years later my weight has stayed the same and I feel great. However, we are all different, we all have natural preferences, and these I believe, must be obeyed. For instance, recently I heard on the radio that some

Eskimos who normally eat a high protein and fat diet had been given a vegetarian diet – it didn't suit them at all. They developed high blood pressure and bad tempers!

Let's go back to why we eat at all. We need food to fuel our bodies and to re-build and repair it. Food gives us energy for living and the correct diet gives us 'Prana' which is the Yoga word for life force. This life force can be added to by taking in fresh food, water, fresh air and sunlight. If we eat heavy, packaged, devitalised foods, our bodies reflect this, whereas if we eat our food in a natural state and as fresh as possible we start to feel alive and well.

When you concentrate on natural foods and obey Yoga's most brilliant piece of advice

'Never more than half fill your stomach with food, leave a quarter for fluid and a quarter for digestion'
HATHA YOGA PRADIPIKA, 58

you will find that gradually you are naturally selecting foods that are going to build health and energy in your body in the correct quantities to keep your body in the best shape for you. We are all made in different shapes and sizes, and each type of body has its own beauty, so accept your body type, learn to love it and live life to the full.

After studying Yoga, many people prefer to become vegetarian and find it suits them perfectly. If so the following healthy eating plan will still be OK,

simply substitute the whole grain rice and pasta dishes for the chicken and fish suggested. Personally, I have tried a vegetarian diet and, quite honestly, it doesn't suit me. I also believe that in a colder climate such as ours a little meat or fish is probably a good thing. Above all, balance is essential. I teach people living a western life who wish to learn Yoga to keep them in good shape, relax and feel healthy. The choice must be an individual one.

'Men who are pure like food which is pure, which gives health, mental power, strength and long life which has taste, is soothing and nourishing and which makes glad the heart of man!'
BHAGAVAD GITA, 17.8

HEALTHY EATING PLAN

Golden Rules for a Slim and Healthy Future

● Eat three meals per day with nothing in between except a fresh fruit snack if a meal is to be delayed

● Never more than half fill your stomach with food, leave a quarter for fluid and a quarter for digestion

● Eat slowly and chew your food thoroughly

● Never eat standing up. This prevents you from nibbling, snacking, eating the kids' leftovers, etc. Many of my pupils have lost over half a stone by employing this rule alone

(If you have allergies or any health problems you must consult your doctor or nutritionist before embarking on the plan.)

Allowances

Drinks: A half-pint of semi-skimmed milk per day, water and herb tea as desired; try to cut down on tea and coffee and have no more than 5 cups per day (if you can cut out tea and coffee totally you might feel considerably better. I was brought up in Nottinghamshire where all problems were solved by putting the kettle on and brewing a nice pot of tea! I love my tea but I do drink it weak with a little milk). You may have 1 glass of wine with dinner, if desired.

Permitted Foods

Fruits – but they must be fresh not tinned or frozen. (One portion = one apple, or one banana, or one orange, or one pear, or one dish of berries, or half a melon, or a large slice of water melon, or half a grapefruit, or two peaches, or four apricots, or four dates, or four plums, or four figs, etc. – every fresh fruit is allowed).

Vegetables – all kinds, as fresh as possible, not frozen or tinned, vary your vegetables as much as you can, have them raw or cooked. All vegetables are allowed except: crisps, chips, butter beans, potatoes or corn on the cob (unless you use the last three as a chicken/fish/rice substitute).

Fish – all sorts, not deep fried, but make it tasty, grilled fish with a little oil or butter or pan fried (always use a non-stick pan). If you have seafood, have it with lemon or a little fresh mayonnaise.

Chicken, poultry, veal or pheasant – all sorts again, roasted, grilled, pan fried, (use a non-stick pan and a very little oil), barbecued, poached, or steam it and serve it with a little sauce (do not deep fry).

Eggs – have as omelettes, scrambled, hard-boiled, etc.

Cheese – either plain or grated cheese, or grilled, as in grilled goat's cheese salad, or use parmesan and enjoy a Caesar salad.

Not Permitted Foods (until you have regained your desired weight) – biscuits, cakes, sweets, buns/bagels, bread (apart from breakfast),chocolate, chips, spirits, jam, soft drinks, canned drinks (except water), hot chocolate, puddings, breakfast cereals.

Do not use diet products, as they may contain additives and preservatives and also 'diet' on the jar makes you feel deprived! Just use natural, normal, healthy food.

Meal Plan

Breakfast
2 pieces of fresh fruit
or 1 piece of fresh fruit and 1 slice of granary toast and a little butter
or 1 piece of fresh fruit and 1 natural yoghurt

Lunch
Main course – 3 oz chicken, turkey *or* fish
or 2 eggs
or 2 oz. cheese
with either large salad plus 1 tablespoon dressing of oil & vinegar or fresh mayonnaise
or 2 cooked vegetables
Dessert – 1 piece of fresh fruit

Dinner
Starter – melon, asparagus or crudities and dip
or clear, homemade soup

Main course – 4 oz fish, chicken, veal *or* turkey
or 2 eggs
or 2 oz cheese,
or small whole grain rice dish or small plate of whole grain pasta
with either 2 vegetables or large salad with 1 tablespoon of dressing

Dessert – 1 piece fresh fruit

Drink – mineral water, *or* 1 glass of wine if desired

There you are. This plan will fit in with your social life, keep you healthy, it is easy to stick to and we have tried and tested it for you. As soon as you have reached your desired weight, stick to the basic plan but increase the portions gradually to maintain your *Fabulous Shape Forever*.

YOGA AND MEDITATION

Meditation is as old as the hills. It is part of all the major religions of the world and is a powerful tool to help us relax, enjoy life to the full and experience wonderful health benefits.

Always remember that you do not have to sit in a full Lotus Position to meditate. Your friendly old armchair will do perfectly well.

Meditation is quite simply sitting in a quiet place, on your own, relaxing and *clearing your mind*. Today life is full of pressure and deadlines. We seem to spend our time rushing from one meeting to another without the time to just sit and BE, to experience and live in the present. Once you learn to take time out, though very difficult at first, the rewards are enormous.

● You start to enjoy the simple things in life which are really around you all the time. For years you might not have had time for these, in your rush to progress in your chosen field. Bird song in the early morning, dew on the grass – such things can give immense pleasure.

'To see a World in a grain of sand,
And Heaven in a wild flower,
Hold Infinity in the palm
   of your hand,
And Eternity in an hour.'

WILLIAM BLAKE

The grass seems greener, the sky seems bluer as you gain a more acute awareness of the present moment.

● You will feel much more positive about your world, your problems will seem to fade and you will frequently receive answers to those seemingly insoluble problems.

'It all depends
On how we look at things
And not how they are themselves.'

CARL JUNG

● Medical research has recently discovered that when we are deeply relaxed chemicals called endorphins are stimulated. These both make you feel great and are very beneficial to the immune system.

'To improve the golden moment of opportunity and catch the good that is within our reach is the great art of life.'

WILLIAM JAMES

● You will experience your own inner peace. The belief in Yoga is 'All we need is within ourselves'.

'Nothing can bring you peace
but yourself. Nothing can
bring you peace but
the triumph of principles.'

RALPH WALDO EMERSON

When we look around we see people rushing around, concentrating on the external world, but our world is made solely by our thoughts. So when we calm down and listen then we experience our true self. We then realise that our happiness is within ourselves. It is how we look at life. We can concentrate on the gloom around us, or quite simply decide to concentrate on the good that is around us. The choice is and always has been our own.

'Not in the clamour of the
   crowded street,
Not in the shouts and plaudits
   of the throng'
But in ourselves are triumph
   and defeat.'

HENRY WADSWORTH LONGFELLOW

How to Meditate

Simply go into a quiet room on your own. Sit with your back straight or lie down. Slow down your breathing and gradually clear your mind. To begin with this is difficult. Thoughts keep crowding in or you fall asleep! But just practice. Sometimes it is helpful to visualise a flower or something beautiful to stop the mind straying. But keep trying – your health and well-being is

159

worth it. Start with five minutes and gradually increase your meditation time to 20 minutes. It is really difficult to control a turbulent mind, but please don't give up. Meditation will not bring us peace – the peace is already inside us, meditation can only help us to find it.

Finally, I do hope you realise by now that Yoga is a brilliant approach to life. The exercises will give you a beautiful healthy body, Yoga breathing will help you relax and give you energy, natural foods will feed your body and keep it in perfect condition and your relaxation and meditation will help you cope with life's stresses and help you experience self realisation.

Remember, it is your life (that might seem crazy, but how often have you spent your time on friends and family but never had time for your self?), learn to enjoy it.

'Do you best to turn your life into a Festival.'

JOHANN WOLFGANG VON GOETHE

'If I had but two loaves of bread
I would sell one and buy hyacinths
for they would feed my soul.'

THE KORAN

In short, fill your life with good books, beautiful music and flowers. Take time to watch the sun set and look at the starry skies. It is up to you to feed your soul the way that food feeds your body.

I send you my very best wishes for your health and happiness.